Outmaneuver Cancer
An Integrative Doctor's Journey

Dr. Robert A. Eslinger, D.O., H.M.D., FAAIM

with Cheryl E. Booth

Printed in the United States of America
First Printing September 2016
ISBN 978-1-48357-646-6

Also by Robert A. Eslinger, D.O., H.M.D.

Chapter 8 of *Defeat Cancer* by Connie Strasheim

DEDICATION

I dedicate this book to my father Lloyd E. Eslinger, D.O. He was an excellent Family Physician and one of the gentlest men I ever knew. A friend to everyone, he always had a joke to share, incorporating humor as part of the healing he offered his patients. He was my inspiration to pursue a career in medicine.

In October 2015, my father passed away at the age of 90. Beloved by his family, friends and patients, he is sorely missed.

***

Not many people read these first few pages in a book but I feel compelled to give credit where credit is due. Therefore I would like to make a second dedication of this book. I would not be here where I am, treating cancer, had it not been for Douglas Brodie, M.D., H.M.D.

He is the one who took away my fear of treating cancer and taught me there is a better way to overcome this devastating disease.

I was privileged to work with him for almost two years before he died right in the office. He was 80 years old and saw patients on the day he died. He always said he wanted to die with his boots on, and he did. He was a giant in the field and an inspiration beyond compare!

DISCLAIMER

This book is not intended as medical advice. It is also not intended to prevent, diagnose, treat or cure disease. Instead, it is intended only to share the research and opinions of the author as well as other doctors who are/were pioneers in the field of medicine, both traditional and integrative, who specialized in cancer research and therapies.

This book is provided for informational and educational purposes only, not as treatment instructions for any disease. Much of the book is a statement of opinion in areas where the facts may be considered controversial.

The book was not written to replace the advice or care of a qualified health care professional. Be sure to check with your own qualified health care provider before beginning any protocols or procedures discussed in this book, or before stopping or altering any diet, lifestyle, or other therapies previously recommended to you by your health care provider.

Cancer treatment is an immensely complex topic and this book should not be regarded as the final word on cancer care. The FDA has not evaluated the statements in this book.

Table of Contents

FOREWORD

My father was Dr. Brodie. He was a venerable giant in the field of alternative medicine and a pioneer in his field. He dedicated his life to his family, his patients and unfolding the knowledge of the human body's ability to heal itself and restore balance. He had the most profound gift of healing, complemented by his incredible bedside manner. He enlightened everyone he touched. He was a fearless man and a steadfast leader.

Dr. Eslinger (Dr. Bob) was "hand-picked" by my father. Dad was inspired by his wealth of knowledge and eagerness to learn the nature of alternative medicine. Dr. Bob, a quick study, was a sponge for this new and different field of medicine. They worked closely together and synergistically developed new, more aggressive protocols.

My father passed away in November of 2005. I have worked with Dr. Bob since that time.

Dr. Bob is at the forefront of a cancer revolution that will change the way people perceive cancer as a "monster" lurking in the darkness. He stands out as one of the most committed, driven, and insightful physicians of this present day. His commitment to finding the highest quality solutions for his patients is second to none.

Always willing to step outside of the proverbial "box," Dr. Bob is never satisfied with merely the status quo; despite the nearly miraculous results he achieves with his patients on a daily basis, he is always looking to refine and improve his protocols. He gives commonsense truths, backed by history and science, which can make an immediate impact on our health, if we take action.

The importance of this book is to unlock the chains that bind you from achieving your optimal health, finding balance and living a long, full life, free from disease.

Marilee Brodie
Patient Liaison, RIMC

PREFACE

I've always liked reading autobiographies and biographical books and stories. Most of the ones that really captured my attention had some great human-interest aspects, of course, so I suppose I should share some of my early background to get the ball rolling. That way you can see how I started out, where my path took me from a young age on through to how I wound up currently running an alternative cancer center in Reno, Nevada.

This book contains lots of reference material to help cancer patients and their families consider new ways of dealing with and overcoming this insidious disease. If that's your primary focus, then great! That was my main motivation in writing it, truthfully. But even if you skip ahead to those sections on nutrition, therapies and other information on cancer that you might not easily find elsewhere, I hope you'll at some point come back and take a little walk down memory lane with me in Chapter One.

I find it fascinating how what people initially think they'll do for a living often has a few bends and turns in the road that we didn't see coming. I've enjoyed most of my forks in the road, and I love what I do for a living. Thanks for reading my book. I want it to leave you with a renewed sense of hope and a heightened awareness of what you can do to demystify and defeat cancer. Information is power, and my hope is that what you'll read here will expand your knowledge on this subject, encourage you to keep doing that through your own continued research, and uplift you and your loved ones along your own journey.

INTRODUCTION

There are a number of key reasons I decided to write this book. I want to do my best to demystify several common unknowns about cancer, including how the disease operates, how to best combat it with integrative medicine while maximizing each patient's overall healing, and educating them about ways to create continued good health.

Unfortunately, Allopathic or conventional Western medicine often lets patients down by leading them to believe there is only one way to treat cancer. In addition, more often than not very little explanation is offered along with the treatment. Sadly, another byproduct of this paradigm is that many doctors are brainwashed into thinking their way is the only way. I'm here to tell you this is not the case!

Here are some of my goals with this book:

1. To share the message that there IS hope for cancer patients. I treat patients diagnosed with any stage of cancer. The way I explain it to my patients is that the therapies we utilize will find and attack the cancer cells wherever they're located. It is absolutely true that Stage 4 is much harder to reverse than Stage 1 of the disease. But those dealing with Stage 4 are certainly not a lost

cause. I frequently say, "None of my patients are incurable. I just don't get to decide who's going to be cured and who's not – but I never know that up front." My job is to do the best I can with all of the knowledge, experience and tools I have at my disposal. I always tell my patients, "There's no such thing as false hope. The time to give up hope is after you take your last breath."

2. I want to do everything in my power to convey to readers the message that integrative/alternative cancer treatment is not some kind of "hocus pocus" – there most definitely is a scientific basis for it.

3. Another important factor to understand is this: cancer is not some type of alien invader whose goal is to infiltrate the body in order to try and kill a person. It is a metabolic disease and when addressed as such, diet is extremely important, among other strategies and treatments. There's an entire chapter (Chapter 5) devoted to diet and nutrition, and this will explain in detail why I say that. So in some ways, having cancer is similar to having diabetes, which is another metabolic disease. In the best protocol to treat diabetes, in part,

you need to use diet to address the problem - it's the same with cancer.

You'll find a number of fascinating books in the Bibliography section, which can serve to further clarify a lot of "mysteries" and unknowns about cancer. My intention in writing this book is to reach the many rather than the few, doing all I can to promote the dissemination of knowledge based upon my almost 40 years of experience as a physician, primarily focusing on the business of what I believe are the most effective ways currently available to kill cancer and heal the person. What follows are some of my credentials in various fields of study, and with a number of organizations.

- ADDITIONAL NOTES: Dr. Eslinger is certified in Family Practice, Osteopathic Manipulation, and a Fellow of the AAIM – American Association of Integrative Medicine. He's also a Founding Member of the IOICP – International Organization of Integrative Cancer Physicians.

He specializes in cancer and chronic disease, and is referred to as an integrative cancer doctor. He is currently licensed to practice medicine in California, Idaho and Nevada.

His present focus is on a specialty in the field known as Biological Medicine, which combines classical treatments with modern science and technology.

Dr. Bob came to Reno in 2004 to work with Dr. Doug Brodie, who was a giant in the field of alternative cancer treatment. Thus began Dr. Bob's career in treating cancer.

In November of 2008, Dr. Bob was appointed to sit on the Board of Homeopathic Medical Examiners for the State of Nevada. More about his credentials and background will be revealed within the contents of this book. For more detail about him, the therapies he practices, or to book a consultation at Reno Integrative Medical Center, visit www.renointegrative.com

- Lindell Eslinger, Dr. Bob's most wonderful wife, made invaluable contributions to this book, and we are extremely grateful for her energy, time and input. In fact, she edited a lot of it, too! Additionally, she writes an extremely informative blog about RIMC and cancer which can be found at http://blog.renointegrative.com

- Dr. Bob also wants to acknowledge the amazing staff of RIMC, and to let them know how much he appreciates the collaborative efforts, energy and skills each of them bring to their work.

Biography of Robert A. Eslinger

Dr. Bob Eslinger was born and raised in Eastern Pennsylvania. After completing his education and training in 1978 he joined the U.S. Public Health Service. At that time it was officially under the Department of the Navy.

He was stationed as the medical director in a clinic located on an Indian reservation 70 miles from the nearest hospital, in Neah Bay, Washington.

After about two months he began noticing that much of what his conventional medical training had taught him just wasn't working, or at least it wasn't working as well as he wanted.

Then he met and started training with one of the local tribal medicine women. He started learning about herbs, supplements and nutrition. This opened a whole new world of healing to him that changed the course of his life. The term "Alternative Medicine" did not even exist at that time.

The internet was only a dream of a few back then, so further training involved reading books and attending conferences. Slowly the concept of "Integrative Medicine" began to take shape in his mind.

After a number of years in private practice, he took a job running a Family Practice and small rural hospital and E.R. in central Idaho. Soon thereafter he became the Medical Director at Cascade Medical Center, a position he held for 13 years.

During that time he began to apply many of the concepts and ideas that are utilized in the practice of Integrative Medicine. His patients loved it, but the hospital board did not.

In 2002 he passed his boards to receive the H.M.D. (Homeopathic Medical Doctor) in the state of Nevada. In 2003 he resigned his position in Idaho, and then worked in a number of E.R.s in rural California before moving to Reno in 2004.

He is licensed to practice medicine in Idaho, California and Nevada. He is certified in Family Practice by the American College of Osteopathic Family Practitioners, and is a Fellow of the American Association of Integrative Medicine. Additionally, he is a Founding Member of the International Organization of Integrative Cancer Physicians.

Dr. Eslinger also sits on the Nevada State Board of Homeopathic Medical Examiners.

Currently he is the owner/medical director of Reno Integrative Medical Center.

Notes from Cheryl E. Booth, co-author

Over the past 30 years I have worked on many books, articles and projects ranging from nonfiction (one of my specialties and favorites, as this book is) to virtually every genre of fiction you might name, as either a ghostwriter, co-author or editor, often wearing multiple hats. Additionally, I've self-published my own books, and am developing a number of screenplays and stage plays, as this amazing book about integrative cancer treatment will be released. If you have, or someone you know has a wonderful story that should be developed and shared with the world, and require assistance with writing and/or editing to get it into print (including print and/or e-book versions), please email Cherylwriter@gmail.com or call 760-808-0170 – I'm always happy to discuss new projects.

I have never been more honored and proud to work on anything, as I am to be a part of *Outmaneuver Cancer*. Dr. Eslinger is truly a gift to this world, and I know that his book will help countless people dealing with cancer. I am thrilled it is getting out there, for I believe in his work beyond the shadow of a doubt. My role has simply been to edit and weave his invaluable message into book form. It is a privilege to be a part of this work, and I'm grateful to be involved.

You may wonder what qualifies me to participate in this book. Other than my writing background, the main reason is because this topic is near and dear to me on a personal level. My beloved mother died from cancer when she was just 54 years of age. I was 15 when she left us, and I found myself faced with assuming the lion's share of caregiving for my younger brother, afflicted with such severe cerebral palsy that he couldn't walk or perform any basic daily needs on his own. Still, he was the most loving and cheerful person I have ever known. I loved him immensely, but coupled with her loss, it was a lot for a teenager to bear. My wonderful father was 15 years her senior, and never expecting to outlive her, he went into an almost impenetrable state of shock for about a year. Thankfully, he came out of it and took over most of Johnny's care, so my last two years of high school were almost "normal."

The point I want to make is this – my mother's first diagnosis was breast cancer, when she was about 48 years old. This was in the late 1960s in the Midwest, and as far as we knew, conventional medicine was the only path. So they performed a radical mastectomy, and then blasted her with cobalt radiation. I still remember the horrific square, blue line scar it left. For awhile, she went into remission, but about 18 months later, cancer cropped up in her uterus and they performed a complete hysterectomy; again, treating her with radiation and other drugs. Relentless as cancer is, particularly in the absence of any integrative medicine being available (or even in our awareness), it persisted and spread even further. My father had to take out a third mortgage to cover medical costs above and beyond any insurance. Eventually he reached the difficult decision to make my mother a ward of the state in order to get her admitted to the only cancer research hospital in Missouri at that time - 90 miles from our home. There were no other options offered or available, and certainly no hope for any improvement was given. She became a human guinea pig for a variety of chemical experimentations (this was 1971, long before we ever heard the word "chemotherapy"), and she went downhill rapidly. Within six months she was gone.

Some of the archaic Western treatment she received is sadly still very much alive and being practiced today. Sure, the methods have been technologically updated, but far too often the results are the same. What Dr. Eslinger practices and teaches is that there is hope far beyond what conventional medicine offers. Hope is something my family never was given, and a boost that we really could have used. I wish integrative cancer therapies had been available for my mother, but "everything happens for a reason" is a philosophy I've adopted over the years. It doesn't make it any easier to accept what takes place sometimes, and losing a dear loved one is something you never quite get over. But the hope and healing that integrative medicine offers are now there for you.

Therefore, whether you're dealing with cancer yourself or are a caregiver or loved one to someone who is, I urge you to read this wonderful book cover to cover. Take it all in, put the dietary and other suggestions into practice, and then call, email or visit Reno Integrative Medical Center for further support and information on the amazing treatment they offer there. Integrative medicine and Dr. Eslinger's vast experience and expertise will make a tremendous difference in your life. The rest of the book is all him – thank you and bless you, Dr. Bob!

In short, Dear Reader, I believe you are about to not only learn much about an integrative approach to cancer, but additionally will find that this book uplifts and inspires you to build/regain hope and faith, and to become as proactive as possible in your healing. I know without question that *Outmaneuver Cancer* will support that on multiple levels – the time has come for this truth to be told.

Cheryl

Chapter 1

Personal Roots

Because readers often like to know some of the background of an author, I will share some of mine with you here. As a doctor working the integrative medical path, I feel it's especially important that you have a sense of how I came to practice medicine in this way.

I grew up in a small town in eastern Pennsylvania. You might say I was born into medicine because my dad, Lloyd Eslinger, was a doctor, and my mom, Doris, was a nurse. Dad was an Osteopathic physician who retired many years ago. He passed away in 2015, after living in a nursing home for some time, due to dementia and other issues. When my mother was 87, being his caregiver eventually reached the point where she simply couldn't handle everything. But she did visit him faithfully every day at the nursing home, and I'm grateful for both their sakes that this was the case.

My dad and I shared a lot of parallels in our lives; so many, in fact, that it seems like more than mere coincidence. I was the second of six children, and in my dad's family of origin, he was also the second-born. I'll go into more detail about other similarities soon, because I believe repeat patterning certainly occurs in many families, and it's just interesting to observe. My father's and mine have definitely given me lots of food for thought through the years.

For right now, though, I'll focus on the medical parallels. For example, I ended up going to the same medical school and interning at the same hospital where he did. He was a D.O., and so am I. That stands for "Doctor of Osteopathic Medicine," as opposed to M.D.s (Medical Doctors), who practice what's known as Allopathic medicine.

Osteopathic physicians receive the exact same training as M.D.s as far as anatomy, physiology, biochemistry, and pharmacology are concerned. Indeed, there are Osteopathic neurosurgeons, gynecologists and pediatricians – every specialist you can imagine. But in addition to all that crossover training, D.O.s also are trained in what's called manipulation - Osteopathic manipulation. In some ways this is similar to what chiropractors do, but there are some differences.

The perspective of Osteopathic medicine entails looking at the whole person instead of just looking at a sick gall bladder, earache or a singular symptom or ailment. Through the years, many of my patients who have gone to M.D.s as well as D.O.s have said that as a general rule, they have found D.O.s tend to be more open-minded than M.D.s. I'll just leave this statement for the reader's consideration by adding that everyone is entitled to his/her opinion. I happen to love being a D.O.

I was in elementary school during the 1960s - the genesis era of the space program. So from grade school on up until my freshman year of high school, I thought I wanted to be an aeronautical engineer and help send astronauts to boldly go where no one before had been. However, once I caught on to how much math was involved in getting an engineering degree, I quickly reconsidered my options. Math was never my close friend!

At some point during my junior year, I applied to college with the redirected focus of getting into a pre-med program. So that's where my personal medical journey began. I was the first student in my high school class to get accepted into college. This was a really big deal at the time, because it was at the height of the Vietnam War, and if you didn't go to college, you went to Vietnam. I'll never forget receiving my acceptance letter in September of my senior year, from the small private college I wanted to attend – Albright College, in eastern Pennsylvania. They closed the letter with a statement that basically said, "Now that you have this acceptance, you can devote your full energy to a successful senior year!" I remember thinking, "Yeah, right! It means it's party time!" Which I suppose is a completely age appropriate response.

My father received his undergrad degree from Muhlenberg College in Allentown, so I purposely chose a different college for my initial university studies. I consciously picked Albright, because I wanted to be a little further away from home. Muhlenberg College and Albright College were definitely competitors in sports teams and all that. But as it turned out my father, my brother and I all went to the same medical school, which is Philadelphia College of Osteopathic Medicine. Interestingly, we all also interned at the same hospital in Allentown.

So now I'd like to examine some of those other parallels between my father and I, because they are many, and to me, at least, they are quite significant. He joined the Marine Corps when he was 19, and when I finished my medical training, I joined the Public Health Service, which was a branch of the Navy. Dad left home and went to the South Pacific whereas I left home and went to the Northwest in Washington State. I'll share more about my time there soon, but for now will focus on more of these father and son parallels.

While I wasn't in a shooting war, my early medical practice started on an Indian reservation, so there certainly is a lot of war history in this region. My father first was in General Practice, identified by the initials "G.P." (General Practitioner). G.P.s treat acute and chronic disease, and provide preventive health care and health education to their patients. Back then there was not yet any such thing as "Family Practice" or a "Primary Care Doctor" designation. So he went into General Practice, and at one time in his career, he was Medical Director of a small hospital in our little town.

Later on in my career, I became the Medical Director of a small hospital in Idaho. I never performed surgery, but Dad did tonsillectomies, and among other things, delivered babies. Even though I never put myself out there as an obstetrician, In my time, I've also delivered babies during emergency births, both on the Indian reservation and in Idaho.

My father was ahead of his time when it came to certain alternative or more holistic medical approaches in many ways. For example, when Nixon "opened up China," as they termed it, and we started hearing about acupuncture more and more in this country, my dad went for acupuncture training and incorporated it into his practice. Another memory that comes to mind is coming home from college on the weekend once to find him laying out all these pills for my mom and himself at breakfast. I asked, "What are those?" and he said, "Oh, these are supplements. You've gotta read about Vitamin E, Vitamin A and Vitamin C…" He was quite enthusiastic about the health benefits they provided.

He was open to that kind of stuff right from the get-go, when it started getting popular. So in his own way, (not as much as I've become) he was definitely alternative medicine-minded, and somewhat of a renegade in that department of medicine. Plus, when he had his first heart attack, he did chelation therapy, and after it helped him, he would tell any of his colleagues in the hospital with heart trouble, "You need to do some chelation – clean out those arteries!" He reported that while some of them went and did it, others said, "I need to check with my cardiologist." He'd reply, "Well, I can tell you what your cardiologist is gonna say," and sure enough, the group that went to their cardiologists didn't end up getting chelation. For years afterward, he said those that wound up getting chelation were still alive, and those that didn't were all dead.

The chelation therapy that he did is an I.V. treatment. In fact, I had a heart attack myself in 2007, and I've done about 75 I.V. chelations. We offer it as one of the therapies in our office now. But with this new energy medicine/quantum physics stuff, we're getting more involved in a process called NES (you'll find more details on this in Chapter 7 about energy medicine). I've come to believe that it's a much gentler way to open up the drainage passageways for heavy metals. I.V. chelation is pretty heavy-handed; it can be hard on the kidneys, so you have to monitor them during the process. So in my own practice, I'm getting a bit away from doing chelation, but it certainly helped my dad.

He used to be a real jokester. When some of his hospital colleagues asked, "Six kids, Lloyd? Why did you have so many?" he would start out by answering, "Oh, because Doris is hard of hearing." Then of course, they'd say, "What does that have to do with it?" and he'd answer, "Well, we go to bed at night, and I'd say, 'You want to go to sleep or what?' and she'd say, 'What?'" Humor goes a long way to help us get through life, as well as when dealing with any kind of illness. I'll address that in this book, too.

My dad and I had another common love, though it expressed itself differently. That is horses. I've always loved to ride them, and have several of my own now. Going to the racetrack, though, fulfilled dad's passion for horses! He used to take Thursdays off from his practice, and Wednesday night after he got off work, he would drive into Allentown and get a copy of *The Morning Telegraph*, the racing form. Then he'd come home, sit in his favorite chair and do all these calculations and formulas based on what he'd read about the horses, the jockeys, owners and all that. He'd go to the track the next day, and he just absolutely loved it. He never rode horses, but connected with them through the racing.

There are other parallels, too; once I made a list of all of them, and there are many. Suffice it to say I basically followed his path, with the exception that when I left medical school, I headed out West. In 1978 after I joined the Public Health Service, I was sent out to the Makah Indian reservation, which is located all the way up on the northwest tip of Washington's Olympic peninsula. It's breathtakingly beautiful, and they have a saying in that neck of the woods that goes, "It only rains once a year – starts in November, and it ends in May." I always tell folks that there's a very good reason it's called the Evergreen State.

The reservation at that time was 70 miles from the nearest hospital, and we didn't have helicopter evacuation, so we had to use an ambulance on a long, winding coastal road. I proceeded to apply all the tools I had learned in my training, but noticed that after a few months of applying those skills, they were often either not working, or not working as well as I wanted. I felt very strongly then, as I do now, that I took an oath to do the very best that I could for every single one of my patients. So I started looking for other solutions, different forms of training and healing. My motto back then became, "I want what works – I don't care where it comes from." That's still my credo today.

At any rate, I was fortunate enough to get to work with a wonderful Makah medicine woman who taught me a lot about supplements, herbs and homeopathics. These were all foreign to me - things of which I had never heard or dreamed. It dawned on me for the first time in my young life that there was this whole world of healing going on out there that I had never been exposed to. Back then, of course, we didn't have the internet, so I had to get books and start studying, in addition to attending lots of conferences. All of this taught me to keep an open mind about a wide variety of therapies. As a general rule, I found that the more natural therapy was far less toxic, and in many cases, the worst that could happen was it wouldn't work. If it didn't, I could slowly, progressively go up the scale of intensity in therapies until hopefully I reached something that worked. I could start with, say, a homeopathic remedy or an herb, and many times I found that in and of itself would help the patient without needing to do something more invasive or that entailed prescription medicine.

Chapter 2

Some Basic Cancer Facts

In the interest of presenting some documented, scientifically proven facts about cancer, it seemed that this chapter was best included at the beginning of the book. The next one is comprised of some of the more recurring questions patients have for me, followed by my answers. But just like the old *Dragnet* TV series, it's always good to start with a simple breakdown of, "just the facts." Some of these facts you may already be well aware of, while others might be new.

Cancer is a Metabolic Disease

What follows is not my own original research – my intent in sharing it is to share and use research that's already been done, and then build upon it from other effective tactics to overcome cancer that I've learned in my own practice.

More and more information is coming to light about this currently, and I'm happy to share what I've learned through this book as well as via speaking engagements. Please feel free to contact me if you belong to an organization that would like more details on booking me as a speaker.

A German doctor named Otto Warburg did excellent research – you can Google him to learn more about his impressive life's work. Dr. Warburg, a German M.D. and Ph.D., received the Nobel Prize in Medicine in 1931 for proving that cancer cells of all types, no matter where they grow, no matter where they spread, have an abnormal way of burning sugar, which is called "anaerobic metabolism." In actuality, the technical name is "anaerobic glycolysis." Please note that they don't issue Nobel Prizes in alternative medicine – Dr. Warburg's was conventional research. One of the primary characteristics of anaerobic metabolism is that it is 18 times less efficient at producing a given amount of energy from a given amount of sugar, and that cancer cells grow without the use of oxygen.

In practical terms, this means that cancer cells require an input of 18 times more sugar on a moment by moment basis than normal cells which use oxygen. Therefore this is the source of the phrase most people have heard that goes, "Cancer loves sugar." Actually, cancer doesn't LOVE sugar; it simply requires 18 times more sugar than normal cells to thrive, because of this anaerobic metabolism. That's why it sucks the sugar out of your system. The other side of the coin is that it's impossible to cure your cancer by not eating sugar, because our brains require sugar at the same level of intensity that they require oxygen. Therefore, if we were to drop your blood sugar to zero, it would most definitely kill the tumor, but would most definitely kill the patient as well.

The way around this dilemma is to gain more knowledge about nutrition (addressed thoroughly in Chapter 5), and to understand that eating highly concentrated sources of sugar – say, anything from a candy bar to pasta, to grains is not a good idea – because all carbohydrates turn into sugar in our body. By eating highly concentrated sources of sugar, or things that convert into sugar, you are essentially throwing gasoline on the fire of the tumor growth. Yet I've heard many more times than you may imagine from lots of patients who come to Reno Integrative Medical Center (referred to hereafter as RIMC) after undergoing conventional Allopathic cancer treatment, that their oncologists have told them, "Oh, it doesn't matter what you eat. You need the calories! You can have milkshakes, ice cream, candy…" In fact, I've heard several times that many oncologists have a big bowl of candy in their waiting room. Some people might call that blatant encouragement of sugar consumption a form of "job security."

When I instruct my patients to ask their oncologist what sugar has to do with tumor growth, however, 99 percent of the time they will say, "Absolutely nothing to do with it." But then they turn right around and order a PET scan, and what that consists of is radioactively tagging sugar molecules, injecting them into the patient's veins, waiting an hour, and then putting them under a nuclear scanner to see where the sugar in the body is concentrated. PET scans are used in conventional oncology every day of the week to discover the location of tumors. And because tumors suck up more sugar than normal tissues, they can pinpoint those tumors using high concentrations of radioactive sugar. Then most turn right around and claim that sugar has nothing to do with tumor growth.

So it's vital to wrap one's mind around the fact that cancer is not to be equated with some "alien invader" that pops up in the body and begins trying to kill the person. It is most assuredly a metabolic disease, as is diabetes. So in addition to the various therapies we offer at RIMC, we also provide instructional information about diet.

There's a wonderful book by Thomas N. Seyfried, PhD titled *Cancer as a Metabolic Disease: On the Origin, Management and Prevention of Cancer.* In this book he expands upon Dr. Warburg's theory that all cancer is a disease of energy metabolism. When you begin to look at it as a metabolic disease, you realize diet plays a major part in addressing the overall situation. When I talk to people about this, they say, "Well, that's very controversial." My reply is, "It's only controversial to people who don't know what they're talking about." Once someone has an understanding of anaerobic metabolism and how cancer needs 18 times more sugar, then there's no controversy at all because that's been tested and proven by conventional medicine.

Apoptosis and Cancer

Apoptosis is a DNA program that's in every one of our normal cells. When a cell is worn out or damaged physically or chemically beyond repair, or has reached an older age where it's not working properly, this apoptosis program takes action. It dwells in what are called the mitochondria in the cell. The mitochondria are the energy furnaces of every single cell. So think of apoptosis this way – when a cell is harmed beyond its ability to heal, whether due to chemical, electrical or physical circumstances, in normal cells apoptosis is triggered and the cell will, in essence, commit suicide, eliminating the old, damaged or worn out cells.

But in cancer cells, apoptosis is specifically turned off, thereby enabling them to thrive, and grow out of control. So even though they're extremely abnormal, they continue growing because this control mechanism has been turned off. We have a means of treating this by use of a protocol called apoptosis enhancement. This will be explained in Chapter 6.

RIMC's Primary Philosophy

Here at the clinic, we like to distill our approach into three simple steps:

1)   Detection

2)   Isolation and

3)   Elimination

Obviously, you first must do everything in your power to detect and identify what type of cancer the patient is dealing with. We also refer to this as de-cloaking – stripping the cancer cells of their armor that is designed to fool the immune system (i.e., turning off apoptosis, using anaerobic metabolism).

The next step is to isolate the cancer cells with our treatment so that it doesn't spread, and follow that isolation up by attacking it. While in attack mode, we utilize therapies that attack the cancer, but simultaneously build up the immune system, so the patient has the best resources to mount that attack. Another way of saying that is, we want to minimize any toxic effects to the normal cells while maximizing the damage to the cancer cells.

I want to clarify something that if you or a loved one is dealing with cancer should take into consideration - cancer does not wait – it grows rapidly. Therefore, the more time you lose by pursuing therapies that in the long run, may cause more harm than good, that's more time for the cancer to grow. So it's of the utmost importance that patients find the correct clinic, one that offers true integrative medicine. This means a combination of both conventional and alternative treatments. We most definitely practice this at RIMC.

You'll read in greater detail about the various therapies and our three-week Boot Camp protocol in Chapter 6, but in this early portion of the book, I wanted to address some of the rudimentary aspects of our mission statement here at Reno Integrative Medical Center.

One of our favorite philosophies is, "Our greatest goal is to promote the healing process so that you can get back to enjoying life again." What follows expands upon that.

RIMC's Clinical Approach

1.   Treat the patient as a whole and not just a symptom. You are not your disease.
2.   Identify, de-cloak and methodically attack the cancer while doing as little harm to the rest of the body as possible.

3. Build the immune system to better assist in the healing process.

4. Provide ongoing support and monitoring both at the clinic, and at home, throughout the healing process.

5. Educate our patients so that they can better care for themselves.

So now that you have a basic description of cancer and how our treatment of it is unique, let's dive into more detail with Q & A in the next chapter.

Chapter 3

Question & Answer Time

Over the years, as you can imagine, I have had a plethora of questions asked of me; some of the same ones have come up several times from a variety of different patients. Since I know the answers are of interest to so many people, I've decided to devote this chapter to those questions and my answers. I hope you benefit from this.

Q: Do you treat all types of cancers?

A: Yes, we do – absolutely.

Q: I've worked my whole life to keep my immune system strong. How is it that I got cancer?

A: Before I start working with you, I do not know the specific triggers that started the cancer, but I can explain how you could develop a tumor in the face of a good, strong, active immune system. That answer is, when a normal cell switches over into the abnormal way that cancer cells have of burning sugar, which is called anaerobic metabolism (burning sugar without using oxygen) at the same time it starts secreting an enzyme called nagalase. We can do a blood test at the clinic to measure the nagalase in your system. The function of nagalase is to seek out and turn off a very specific cell in your immune system called the macrophage cell. The macrophage cell's major job is to find and eliminate abnormal cells in the body. So when it's turned off by the nagalase, I call it "cloaking" of the tumor to detection by the immune system.

We universally see elevated nagalase levels in the blood of cancer patients when there's a tumor present. So that's how you could have a good, strong, functioning immune system, but the cancer has figured out a way to "cloak" itself from detection by the immune system. And then we utilize a specific therapy called GcMAF – the MAF stands for Macrophage Activating Factor. This is a tiny injection given twice a week, and it goes in and reactivates the macrophage cells. The one thing that must be present for the GcMAF process to work is that the person must have adequate levels of Vitamin D in their system. This will be addressed in greater detail in Chapter 6, which covers therapies done at the clinic.

Q: So is the Vitamin D level subject to the individual and their needs?

A: Yes, it is. Currently, it's a known fact in this country that the vast majority of people have very low Vitamin D levels, because Vitamin D is what your body – specifically your skin – can manufacture when exposed to sunlight. But in modern times, everyone's been taught to be afraid of too much sunlight. It didn't used to be that way. Today people either don't get exposed to sunlight, or they heavily use sunscreen to prevent skin cancer. So we supplement with an emulsified version of Vitamin D that are sublingual drops (which go under the tongue). This is after doing blood tests for Vitamin D levels to tell if the person has an adequate level.

It should be noted that many times people who are always out gardening, tanning, and doing other activities that place them out in the sun frequently, are shocked to find out their Vitamin D levels are low. So there are a number of contributing factors to this deficiency, and we want to boost the individual's system to the proper level.

Q: If someone's been a smoker pretty much all their life and simply doesn't really want to quit, not altogether, anyway, what do you tell them?

A: I tell them that whatever they do with their body is their choice, their decision. But it's an established fact that smoking will slow down healing from any disease. And in fact, even conventional surgeons know that if someone requires surgery and they continue to smoke, they're going to be a much slower healer than someone who's a nonsmoker, because that's been proven; it's a scientifically, medically proven fact. So I would say to them, "It's up to you if you choose to continue smoking, but realize you are hampering your immune system and your overall bodily systems from healing from ANY disease, and in particular from cancer. So if you want to stack the cards against yourself, go ahead and continue to smoke."

Q: Why doesn't my insurance pay for your treatment?

A: That's an excellent question, and one that might best be posed to your insurance company. Any therapies out there, which are, quote "natural," are not patentable, and if it's not patentable, nobody can make lots of money from it.

More often than not, your insurance company is going to give you an answer along the lines of, "Well, those are not 'approved' therapies," and then if you want to delve further, you could do some research on your own to determine 'approved by whom?' The short answer with regard to natural products or therapies is that they are not patentable, and companies are not interested in developing studies to prove if they're effective or not if they don't have a guarantee of multi-dollars at the end of that study. So the reason we don't accept insurance in our office is because they don't cover most of the therapies that we do – they simply won't pay for them.

Q: Why don't I hear about this from my doctor, or in magazines and on TV?

A: This ties into the previous answer, and will require some due diligence on the reader's part to get all of the facts. Most conventional doctors are either unwilling or afraid to "think outside the box" because it's a very real possibility that their licenses would be threatened. Here in Nevada where the clinic is located, I'm in a very unique situation because of the protection that we have in this state to practice alternative medicine. Currently the only three states in the U.S. that allow the practice of alternative medicine are Nevada, Arizona and Connecticut.

Another part of the answer is that people can find information on these therapies, but they have to search for it on the internet. This is problematic, because in many ways, the internet is both a blessing and a curse. I say that because anybody can put anything on the internet. For example, they could post a radical claim such as, "I cured my cancer by making a tea from horse poop!" So you find a really mixed bag of therapies and claims online, some ludicrous and some legit.

When you start investigating alternative therapies, some outrageous claims could very well pop up with no backing from any medically trained people. And when someone has no medical training, they have no idea how to "separate the wheat from the chaff" – so that's the downside of the internet. The upside for me is that I can go on the internet and research some of the latest studies that are going on in Germany, say, with mistletoe. Those are available online as well, and that's the blessing of the internet. So the thing that people have to realize is they must find a professional that they trust.

I'll give one specific example of the downside. When Dr. Brodie was still alive, we actually had an email that came in through our website saying, "Please thank Dr. Brodie for all of his recommendations on fighting cancer. I did all of them." Well, we were horrified that someone attempted to self-treat in the extreme like that, with no professional medical supervision to monitor and administer proper dosages and so forth. That was proof positive many people will go to extremes to look for ways to not have to come to a clinic like ours, and do things at home, oftentimes using so-called "remedies and cures" they find online which aren't based on scientific fact. The treatment we offer is all based on science. You most definitely want a licensed physician overseeing your cancer treatment – that's why I'm here.

Q: If you are alternative and integrative, why do you use chemos? Aren't they bad for you? I keep hearing and reading that it's poison and so harmful.

A: While we do use conventional chemo drugs, it is in a very targeted manner - we use 90 percent less than a full dose of chemo. This is done via IPT therapy, and you'll find a detailed explanation in Chapter 6 of that. Basically, it involves the use of insulin to drop the blood sugar and make the cancer cells much more susceptible to the chemos. By doing so, there's a very strong likelihood of killing them without harming the immune system and the other systems in the body. So that's a perfect example of integrative medicine utilizing things from conventional medicine that have a time and place, if properly utilized.

In 2006, I quit using chemo in IPT for an entire year, and our success rate dropped significantly. When I shifted back to using chemos at 10 percent in this IPT therapy, our success rate went back up again. So as of this date, I have not found anything that I can substitute for the specific job that the chemos perform in an IPT treatment for treating cancer. I most certainly do not condone the use of full dose chemo. So for right now, I consider the 10 percent solution a necessary evil in order to do the best possible job for my patients. When something else is discovered that is medically and scientifically proven to work as well, I'll gladly stop using it altogether.

Q: Why can't you treat anybody under 18?

A: While the fact of the matter is that I can treat young people and children under the age of 18, I choose not to. It's controversial enough to treat adults with alternative medicine for cancer in this country, but using it to treat children currently is not only frowned upon but also actively resisted by the legal system, as well as the medical system. There have been documented cases in other states where parents of a child diagnosed with cancer do not want to have full dose chemo or radiation given to that child, instead wanting to choose alternative medicine, they are told by the "powers that be" that if they do, the state will come in and take not only the child being treated away from them, but all the rest of their children, too, because it will be declared they are performing child abuse. Some of those states have followed through with this extreme measure and taken children away from the parents, and then forced the child with cancer to do full dose chemo.

If you'd like to learn more about this horrifying fact, there's a documentary titled *Cut, Poison, Burn*. In this film, they follow a family that happened to. Sadly, the boy ends up dying from the chemo, not the cancer. Search *Cut, Poison, Burn* on YouTube and you'll find excerpts from the documentary.

And just a quick side note – on the label of chemo meds it even says, "Do not give to children."

Q: I read on the internet that I should alkalinize my water. Will that help cure my cancer?

A: The short answer is NO. To give more in depth insight, I need to explain that as mentioned before, there's a lot of misunderstood or misinterpreted information posted online by people without medical training. Some practitioners teach that if the body becomes too acidic, that will cause cancer. The actual fact supported by scientific basis is that the acidity is caused by cancer. It's not the trigger causing the cancer; it's the result of the cancer. This is because of that abnormal anaerobic metabolism mentioned throughout this book.

In short, anaerobic metabolism is how cancer cells burn sugar - without using oxygen. This process has one very large waste product, and that is lactic acid. Lactic acid is normal in a human body, but when this happens due to the cancer cells' metabolism, there are much larger amounts of it around the cancer cells, in their immediate environment. Therefore it's the result of the cancer metabolism – not the cause of the cancer to begin with. So no - you cannot cure cancer by neutralizing the acidic environment.

It does make sense to try and keep the pH levels close to neutral in the human body (pH is the scale or the measure of acid versus alkaline). But it is also compounded by, or complicated by the fact that it's imperative for the pH of the blood in the body to swing back and forth between acid and alkaline throughout any given day in order to perform all the functions of the human body. You'll find more specific information on this in the "Water" section of Chapter 5 of this book, much of it based on the work of an amazing Romanian physician named Emanuel Revici. So please read or reread that chapter, if you're seeking more facts about this.

Q: Why is cancer such a fast-growing disease?
A: Not all cancers are fast-growing, but that is true of the majority of tumors. Again, the reason is this anaerobic metabolism, which has a much higher burn rate than conventional metabolism. That's why thermogram testing is valuable as a screening tool to find things like breast cancer or thyroid cancer, because the cancer as a general rule will be hotter than the surrounding tissue. Due to that higher rate of

metabolism, a faster rate of cell division occurs; in other words, the faster the cell division, the faster the cancer grows.

There is a process called apoptosis that I discussed in detail in the preceding chapter titled "Some Basic Cancer Facts." But because we tend to retain and learn through repetition, here's a quick refresher – apoptosis is a DNA program that's in every one of our normal cells. When a cell is worn out or damaged physically or chemically beyond repair, or has reached an older age where it's not working properly, apoptosis gets turned on in those old, damaged or worn out cells. Its job is to basically cause the damaged cell to commit suicide. But apoptosis is specifically turned off in cancer cells, so that is why they grow out of control. Even though they are very abnormal, they keep growing and getting bigger because this control mechanism has been turned off.

Q: Do you have a way of changing that?

A: We do have some specific components of our therapy that can be utilized to reignite this apoptosis process. One is called DCA, or dichloroacetate, and the other is called butyric acid, or butyrate. Butyrate is the salt of butyric acid, and it is made from dairy products. It will also work in the same way as DCA, reigniting this apoptosis process. A third component is oxaloacetate. All of these are in capsule form, so are taken orally.

Q: My doctor says that I can eat anything, like lots of fruit, just as long as I'm eating high calories to keep weight on me. Is that true?

A: Many cancer patients are told by their oncologists that they can eat whatever they want, and are frequently also told that sugar has absolutely nothing to do with tumor growth. That is 180-degrees exactly opposite of the truth. The truth is that sugars will feed tumor growth; consumption of high concentrations of sugar is like throwing gasoline on a fire.

The reason is this anaerobic metabolism that I keep going back to – this burning of sugar without using oxygen. I already mentioned how anaerobic metabolism has a much higher rate of burn than normal metabolism, and that's why it puts out more heat. So that's why I recommend a Ketogenic diet, which is extensively covered in Chapter 5.

Q: Will you treat someone who is in Stage 4, or is there a certain stage where you recommend they go elsewhere for treatment rather than coming to the clinic?

A: I generally pay very little attention to the stage, because I have absolutely worked with Stage 4 cancer patients, and there is no Stage 5. What conventional oncologists pretty much universally tell patients is, "Stage 4 cancer is incurable." I tell my patients that the reason oncologists say that, is because they've never seen *their* therapies work with it. I HAVE, using integrative medicine. I have seen Stage 4 patients reverse the cancer. Again, I tell patients, "Once you've seen that happen one time, and I've seen it more than once, you can no longer make that statement." So all the staging process means is that Stage 1 is a local tumor; Stage 2 is localized spread to adjacent tissues; Stage 3 has spread to whatever that area's lymph nodes are; and Stage 4 has spread across the diaphragm to another body cavity.

The therapies we utilize will find and attack the cancer cells wherever they're located. It is true that Stage 4 is much harder to reverse than Stage 1 of the disease. But those patients are not a lost cause. I say, "None of my patients are incurable. I just don't get to decide who's going to be cured and who's not – but I never know that up front." So my job is to do the best I can with what I have and tell my patients, "there's no such thing as false hope," and that the time to give up hope is after you take your last breath.

Q: I've read that cesium is a good therapy for cancer - do you do it?

A: Cesium is a very alkalizing mineral that is taken out of the earth, and there is a contingent of people out there that claim to have allegedly cured cancer by administering cesium doses to cancer patients. I utilized cesium therapy, or what's called "high pH" or "alkalization therapy" for a full year back in 2006. In my experience, it does not work. What happened in my situation is that we would administer intravenous and oral cesium to patients, and I can guarantee it does raise the pH of the blood and the urine, and make it much more alkaline.

The problem is that the one place you have to be very acidic is your stomach. We universally found that when we would really metabolically push someone until their urine pH was higher than a pH scale reading of 8.0, every single one of them started to vomit and experience diarrhea with undigested food in it, and that wasn't the only thing. If that had been the worst thing but the cancers still went away, I would still be doing that treatment. But the cancer did not go away even at that alkaline level, so we ultimately stopped using cesium altogether.

Q: Why can't I get IPT treatments in the hospital?
A: My short answer is twofold – one, why don't you ask *them* that? And two, they don't know about it because they've never been taught about it. You have to do some digging, some investigation, and you also have to understand the physiologic nature of cancer, and the anaerobic metabolism that's involved with it, i.e., that need for 18 times the normal amount of sugar – you have to comprehend all of that in order to understand that IPT makes total sense when trying to address cancer. So if you have either forgotten or ignored those portions of your medical training to the point where you don't understand the physiology of cancer and its needs, then you don't comprehend the need for something like IPT. Conventional medicine does

not train their doctors about IPT. So that's why it's not being administered in hospitals.

The other question that goes along with that is, patients say, "Well, if it's so effective, why isn't it being done in hospitals?" and the reason is what I touched upon earlier – it would require the pharmaceutical industry manufacturing 90 percent less quantity of the chemos than they are right now, which I doubt is going to happen anytime soon.

Q: High dose Vitamin C is listed as one of your therapies. Can I just take a lot of Vitamin C tablets at home? Is it the same?

A: It is definitely not the same. When it's true high dose Vitamin C, it's actually in a category of therapies called oxidative therapies (See Chapter 6 for more details); this includes the use of ozone, which is a form of oxygen, and also intravenous hydrogen peroxide. When I say, "high dose Vitamin C" – I mean at least higher than 10 grams a day, and our usual dose of I.V. Vitamin C is between 50 and 75 grams, which is 50 to 75,000 milligrams. Usually a single Vitamin C tablet is either 500 milligrams or 1,000 milligrams, which is one gram. If you approach an oral dose over 10 grams a day, or 10,000 milligrams, the vast majority of people will end up having diarrhea from that dosage. So they can't continue higher doses than that and tolerate it, because of the diarrhea.

Now, even though Vitamin C itself is an antioxidant, above 10,000 milligrams or 10 grams a day it becomes an oxidative therapy, because it enables a certain type of white blood cell in our system to produce more hydrogen peroxide internally. So it becomes an oxidative therapy. Oxidative therapies as a general rule can be very helpful in addressing cancer because not only does cancer not like oxygen, but too much oxygen can be deadly to cancer cells.

Q: Do you have a therapy that can put high oxygen into the body to kill the cancer? Is that a possibility?

A: Yes, we do. And that is the category of therapies I just mentioned – by using oxygen in a certain combination, or what we call the oxidative protocol – we utilize ozone gas, hydrogen peroxide and high dose Vitamin C, as well as administering medical grade oxygen through breathing, and not all at the same time. But it's a specific order of a protocol.

Now, the way the ozone is administered, it can be given direct intravenous; it can also be mixed in with a sample of the blood taken out and mixed into sterile saline or salt water solution, and then run back in through a chamber surrounded by ultraviolet light bulbs; that therapy is called UBI – Ultraviolet Blood Irradiation. It triggers an oxidative reaction in the blood, so the use of these different therapies result in much higher doses of oxygen in the body than what would normally be there.

Now, there is also a question about what is called "hyperbaric oxygen therapy," and this is the treatment where someone lies down inside a sealed chamber; then the chamber is pressurized, filled with 100 percent oxygen, and they stay in there for set periods of time. Some doctors utilize hyperbaric treatment for cancer. It is a specific form of oxidative treatment; however, I do not use it at the clinic. Instead, we use five different forms of oxidative therapies, which are described in Chapter 6, titled *Boot Camp & Various Therapies.*

Q: You say you have a "Boot Camp" for patients to attend for 3 weeks – why 3 weeks?

A: The three weeks we utilize is 5 days a week for 3 weeks and Dr. Doug Brodie originated it; he's the doctor I came to Reno to work with originally, and I continued doing that same principle. Now, that being said, there are some protocols around the country, and even in Mexico in clinics where they treat cancer; most of them utilize the three-week time period. Now, the concept to understand is that we never tell people the cancer will be cured within 3 weeks and it'll be gone.

There's a concept called a "critical threshold" and those 3 weeks of Boot Camp allow enough time to start the healing process. So we view that 3-week time period as the critical threshold, followed by instructing patients on how continue with different therapies at home. We also have our patients return to our clinic for 3 to 5 days once a month after the end of Boot Camp, until we can verify that the cancer is resolved. Please refer to the "Boot Camp" chapter (Chapter 6) in this book and/or to our website www.renointegrative.com for more complete details.

Chapter 4
Cancer and Fear

I've come to believe that one of the very biggest things for any cancer patient, as well as their families, is to overcome the huge fear factor that's involved with their initial cancer diagnosis. We do everything in our power at the clinic to lessen that fear, and it's my sincerest hope that this book will go a long way towards doing that on a much larger scale.

Basically put, fear stimulates the sympathetic overdrive, which depresses the immune system. Personally, I maintain that any doctor that uses fear to get their patients to do their therapies is in violation of their Hippocratic oath. The reason I feel this way is because all doctors – whether naturopathic, D.O.s, or Western medicine/Allopathic M.D.s have all been taught these same principles – this is not exclusive to me. Then the majority of them have proceeded to forget those tenets and principles. In my experience, I've observed that every medical school in this country, during the first six months of training, teaches all students how we are each biochemically and physiologically unique. Then they spend the next eight-and-a-half years teaching them how to treat everybody the same way. It's such hypocrisy, yet most doctors never address it.

It's never in a patient's best interest when on the path to healing to be treated in a "one size fits all" type of standardization. Human beings are simply not geared that way. We're not some sort of robotic reproductions or clones who have interchangeable parts and needs – at least not yet! We're far from being just standardized objects on some type of assembly line that can be treated universally. Everyone's unique, and body, mind and spirit all play important roles in health. That's one of the basic principles of PNI, which stands for psychoneuroimmunology, a whole new field in conventional medicine.

One of the main missions for me as a doctor is to help treat patients in every beneficial way possible, while simultaneously assisting them in overcoming fear and replacing it with hope.

It's fairly common when someone first comes in that they obviously feel very petrified. When I ask, "What are you afraid of?" the most common answer is, "I'm gonna die." My first response is, "Well, we're all gonna die – that's not a question of 'if' – it's a question of 'when.' And it has far more to do with the quality of the days that you have here as opposed to the number of days." So we discuss this further, and everyone agrees that they don't want to live to be 120, drooling into their lap in a rocking chair in a nursing home. But normally people think of death as far off in the nebulous future somewhere, further away. Getting a cancer diagnosis brings it right up close and personal, and then the follow-up fear which sets in is based upon things they've either witnessed themselves, or heard about patients having gone through during conventional treatment. Some of these include loss of body function, in some cases no longer being able to take care of themselves; weight loss, severe pain, nausea and vomiting, diarrhea – all of those things serve to create even more fear.

So obviously, when it comes to the fear about conventional treatment, that's an easy one to help them calm down about because we don't do conventional treatment. I explain to them in as much detail as they can handle about the different options we have to treat the cancer, without causing those scary, negative results. Granted, some of our patients develop nausea, diarrhea or pain, but that's why I practice what I call integrative cancer treatment. Simply put, I administer therapy that can help with those problems. The therapies would include starting off with gentle things like herbs or homeopathic remedies to deal with those problems, and if those don't work, then on up to and including the use of prescription medication for pain, nausea or diarrhea, if need be. This is why I maintain that unless a doctor has a full practice license, training and experience in both alternative and conventional medicine, they can't do truly integrative cancer treatment, because what are they integrating? It takes a long, long time for a physician to truly become trained and experienced in integrative treatment. But I believe what it has to offer is the best of both worlds;

therefore I believe integrative treatment is the way to go, and that's why I practice what I practice.

Regarding specific fears, I go beyond talking only about fears with many patients, and delve into discussing potential triggers that could have started the tumor growing, or set the stage for the tumor to grow. Let me give you an example based on the work of Dr. Gerhardt Hamer in German New Medicine.

Hamer was a certified oncologist in Germany who was treating cancer patients with chemo back in the 1980s, when his 19-year-old son was shot and killed. Due to his horrific shock, grief and loss, he subsequently developed testicular cancer himself. He wondered if that trigger could have set the stage for the process of the tumor growing. So he began asking his patients what kinds of stresses they experienced in their lives within the two to three years right before their diagnosis, and he started getting some amazing answers. Through this, he developed a whole system of evaluation, which he calls "conflict shock." This encompasses mental, emotional, and psychological shock that hits somebody and virtually blindsides him/her; it's something totally unexpected which catches them off-guard and really hits them hard.

Then he started making correlations with different kinds of cancers in different organs with different kinds of conflict shock. Sadly, what happened was they locked him up, put him in jail. But he refused to allow that to stop him; he kept teaching from jail. He had his students come visit him and he'd give them notes, and they would teach classes. When he got out of prison in Germany, he left and went to France. Eventually the French authorities began hounding him and he ended up going to Spain. Finally, he left Spain because the German Attorney General was trying to extradite him back to Germany to go back in prison for another five years for the crime of "inciting the public..."

All of this due to the fact that he teaches principles contrary to the conventionally accepted ideas of what causes cancer. After learning about all that he has endured as well as many other travesties others have suffered, I've been known to say, "The Inquisition is not dead, it's alive and well in modern medicine." I believe Dr. Hamer is currently in Finland under political asylum. He's in his late 70s, so he's probably going to stay there in order to avoid going back to Germany and jail. I share his story here because I believe his research is incredibly valid about the kinds of things that contribute to the overall stress situation that can add to the fear. One specific example that he cites regarding cancer of the liver is that it is associated with a person's loss of sustenance. Now, these things are totally a personal interpretation.

Someone's loss of sustenance could be physical, it could be emotional, it could be financial - all are contributors.

Another big example he gives is that pancreatic cancer is what I have come to term as a "frustrated entitlement." He says many times it has to do with family inheritance.

An interesting little story along these lines is about a patient of mine a few years ago that came in with liver cancer. As I was explaining these principles to him, specifically about pancreatic cancer, he almost fell out of his chair. I could tell he was startled, and he said, "How did you know that?" I replied, "I'm just telling you what Dr. Hamer says." He then went on to tell me a story about how his mother had died a few years prior to that, and the only siblings were he and his sister. When his mother died, he was married and his sister was not. He said to his sister, "I'd like to have Mom's wedding ring, and you can have the engagement ring." But his sister said, "No! I'm entitled to both the rings – I want both rings!" She proceeded to fight him in court, up to and including a trial, which she lost. Two years later she was diagnosed with pancreatic cancer and after that, she was dead. So that is a pretty clear example of what I'm talking about.

What the overall effect of this whole thing is, the fear of dying and all these bad symptoms as well as the stress caused by these conflict shocks; the end result is what I call "sympathetic overdrive." Now, sympathetic overdrive is a term that describes what's happening in the autonomic nervous system. Every human being has two nervous systems – the central nervous system is the brain and the spinal cord, as well as all the nerves that we think, move and feel with; whereas the autonomic nervous system is the system that runs everything that's on automatic. These are functions you don't have to think about. If you had to think about everything like your heartbeat and breathing rate, you'd never be able to do anything else. So those are handled by the autonomic nervous system and it's divided into two parts – the sympathetic and the parasympathetic.

The sympathetic system is the classic "fight, flight or fright" reaction – it's the adrenaline rush when you get scared or perceive that you're in a dangerous situation. It's designed to help you save your personal existence; it shifts you into overdrive so that you can run faster, jump higher, be stronger – it's the system that allows a grandma to pick up the car that rolled backwards down the driveway and landed on her grandson. That's called sympathetic overdrive, and the good thing about it is, it works. It has saved countless people's lives in life-threatening situations. The downside is that when you shift into sympathetic overdrive, which is a reflex, it's not a conscious decision - it happens automatically. Your subconscious determines whether you're going to shift into that. When that happens, your subconscious also determines which systems in the body are not essential to immediate survival. The two systems in your body at the top of that list are your immune system and the digestive system. Of course, your immune system is your major ally in protecting you from all kinds of diseases, but in this situation - needing to fight abnormal cancer cells – the digestive system feeds the immune system, providing energy to it. So without these two systems heavily online, you've got a big problem! I mean, for the next 10 minutes, you can survive without either of these two systems very easily. But stretched out over the next 10 days, or 10 weeks – you've got a big problem.

So I maintain that any doctor who uses fear to try to get a patient to do their therapy has just automatically violated their Hippocratic oath, because they have hampered their patient's immune system and their ability to heal from ANY disease. I've heard many times of oncologists who tell patients, "You have to do this chemo or you're gonna die." That handicaps the patient right out of the starting gate. So this is a big reason to deal directly with these issues, because if you don't, you're hampering the immune and the digestive systems, and the therapies will never work as well as they could.

So first of all, the way we help people begin to deal with this is to talk with them about how essential it is to engage in some sort of activity that they love to do. Anything from a hobby like knitting to just about anything; it could even be doing deep breathing exercises. But they need to find some sort of activity to trigger what's called "the relaxation response," because it pushes us into what's called parasympathetic overdrive, which is the exact opposite of the sympathetic overdrive. So I tell them, "When you say, 'Oh, honey – look at the beautiful sunset...' or 'smell those beautiful roses...' that's when your body takes a big sigh and your brain goes, 'Okay, now we can relax.'" This is the point where your immune system starts to approach maximum strength.

So any activity someone enjoys that relaxes him/her is going to trigger that response. For example, it can be a specific exercise, an activity, or going to a specific place...I add that because when patients come to work with us at RIMC, I always suggest if they have a car, sometime while they're here they should drive up Mount Rose Highway. Over the top of the mountain, partway down the other side there's a pullout – a lookout over the other side of the mountain where you can see all of Lake Tahoe from one place. It's what I call an alpha view, because I believe it triggers alpha brainwaves, which is what you go into when you're completely relaxed. So I suggest taking in a beautiful view whenever possible.

We have a tool in the office we use called an "insight CD" that requires wearing headphones or ear buds - you can Google this yourself - just search "insight CD" and it'll pop right up. They've done a bunch of research with this; it's a tool used to synchronize the two hemispheres of your brain. In a nutshell, the definition of two sides of the brain for most people breaks down this way: the left side is the scientific "just the facts, ma'am," while the right side sees sizes, shapes, sunsets, colors and so forth. These two hemispheres rarely are working with each other; usually we jump back and forth very rapidly between them, and typically one is in dominance.

You can usually tell just by looking at or talking to somebody which hemisphere they're operating in, but this insight CD plays two versions of a specific sound. For example, one sound might be heavy rainfall on a blacktop parking lot, and the other one is ocean waves, surf. But imbedded underneath these sounds are two frequencies; one goes into one ear, and a slightly different frequency goes into the other ear. The brain is always trying to look for a connection pattern, and the frequency going into your right ear goes into the right hemisphere as well as into the left hemisphere to help create that pattern. This CD has three 20-minute tracks on it, and eventually you can hear that sound. But in the beginning you can't, you just hear the overlying sound.

What happens is, your brain creates what's called a harmonic, a combination of those two different frequencies. At one point, both hemispheres start vibrating at the harmonic frequency. You can read from the research on their website that when both sides of your brain start vibrating at the same frequency together, it pushes you into parasympathetic overdrive. So it's a very healing experience – it's kind of like being a yogic monk for 30 years, only you get to experience it in the first hour! So it's a great tool. People can listen to it while doing almost anything else – we don't recommend doing it while you're driving. But if they're just sitting there getting an I.V., they can listen to this and receive the therapeutic benefit. It's also referred to as hemi-sync.

The NES System and Energy Medicine

I go into more depth about the NES System in Chapter 7 (Energy Medicine) and there you'll read more about how it addresses the emotions. Interestingly enough, it has incorporated into the evaluation process many – not all – of the points that come up on the evaluation; many times it will give what they call the "body/mind connection." It actually incorporates a lot of Hamer information, where it assesses that "this person has experienced a financial trauma somewhere in their past," or something along those lines. I've had patients just be astonished, asking, "How does it know that?"

It doesn't happen every time, unfortunately, but on a regular basis people's jaws just drop at what this report comes up with; things they've never brought up in conversation with me, but after it comes up on the computer they start describing some major trauma they've been through, either as a child or a few years prior. They don't see any connection between that and what their problem is but there IS a connection. So it's really exciting stuff.

Also, humor is truly a powerful ally in creating healing. I remember a long time ago reading Norman Cousins' book *Anatomy of an Illness*, about using humor and laughter as a tool to overcome disease. I don't necessarily talk to my patients a lot about humor, I just joke around with them a lot myself; my Dad used to do the same thing, and because he was my role model I tend to follow suit. I do believe it would be a good idea to get a series of comedies on Netflix or DVDs, sit down, and enjoy a comedy movie marathon. In India, there are clinics where they do laughing therapy. Groups of people get together and the therapists usually have very funny laughs; they basically just stand around in a circle and the therapist starts laughing; pretty soon everyone is laughing. They laugh for a set period of time, and it's not only the humor, it's the breathing that's involved with it that contributes to the healing - endorphins being released and so on. I think that's a much under-appreciated tool.

Chapter 5

The Importance of Healthy Nutrition

Cancer's Sugar Connection

Since my goal with this book is to demystify and outmaneuver cancer, this topic is a critical key point. I would say that almost 99 percent of people that I see as cancer patients tell me when they first come in that they've heard the phrase, "cancer loves sugar." So one of their first responses to that prior to working with me is to decide, "Well, I'll just stop eating sugar." While I think that's a good idea is some regards, it's impossible to cure cancer by not consuming sugar, because our brains require sugar on the same level of intensity that they require oxygen.

As pointed out in the first chapter, cancer is a metabolic disease, just as diabetes is a metabolic disease. So I explain to patients about sugar consumption along these lines, "I can give you a high dose of insulin, drop your blood sugar to zero and yes, it would kill the tumor, but it would kill you, too." Understandably, most patients don't consider that to be a successful outcome! Just as you read earlier in this book, the fact is that cancer doesn't *love* sugar. Cancer *requires* 18 times more sugar than normal cells because of its anaerobic metabolism. Dr. Otto Warburg proved this scientifically, and in fact, won the Nobel Prize for his work on this subject.

Cancer's relationship with sugar has already been addressed in Chapter 2 ("Some Basic Cancer Facts"). Please refer back to it, if you feel the need to revisit that topic. Now, let's move on and explore some other nutrition issues.

Everything in Moderation – Including Moderation!

I encourage my patients not to go off of the deep end about anything. Becoming fanatical about things can certainly have its share of cons, not just pros. For example, consider the controversy about microwave ovens. Some people really go overboard about this, refusing to even set foot in a home that has a microwave, whether it's currently in use or not! Personally, I use a microwave oven intermittently, usually just to reheat leftovers, things like that, if I'm in a hurry.

Balance in all things is a great goal. Overall, I tell my patients, "Moderation in all things, including moderation." I also tell them, "Human beings without treats die of boredom." So I always use the example of chocolate cake, because I LOVE chocolate cake. I tell them, "If you love chocolate cake, and you come see me and I say, 'Oh, you can't have chocolate cake ever again in your life because you have cancer,'" then naturally, what's their brain going to scream for? Chocolate cake.

This is the same principle that I've used many times to help people stop smoking, or shift away from other unhealthy habits. The basic premise is, you set a time frame, and tell yourself, "Okay, you're allowed to have a small piece of chocolate cake every two weeks." So if you're walking by the local bakery and you smell and see a chocolate cake and your brain starts screaming for it, you just say to yourself, "Oh, yeah – we talked about that. I can have a piece of chocolate cake, and it'll be in a week and a half." Then your brain goes, "Okay, if I know it's coming, then I can relax," and the craving will tend to go away. But then what you're required to do, and sometimes I even write out a prescription for this – you're required to absolutely eat that piece of chocolate cake in a week-and-a-half, and you're mandated by doctor's orders to enjoy it! Because if you're sitting there eating it, and thinking, "Oh, man, this is terrible for me, I know it. But it tastes SO good!" - then it's going to be horrible for you. That's a basic self-fulfilling prophecy, and you're just setting yourself up to fail or have a really bad experience, plus a guilt trip – who needs one of those? It's vital to set your brain up as a tool that helps you, rather than one that fights with you.

In general when it comes to the dietary side of things, I believe that human beings were meant to be omnivores. Personally, from what I've observed about it many times over, I do not believe vegetarianism is a healthy lifestyle. I have to say that 95 percent of the vegetarians that I have seen as patients are not healthy people. They still do get cancer, and I have trouble keeping their protein and hemoglobin levels up. I believe this is because humans are meant to be omnivores, who by definition eat a little bit of everything. I was married to a vegetarian for eight years back in the 1980s, and in my experience, most vegetarians have that diet for philosophical reasons – usually it distills down to the fact that they don't want to harm the animals. While that's lovely and commendable, I give them a dose of reality by saying, "Your physiology doesn't give a hoot about your philosophy, and your physiology is basically the same as it was thousands of years ago." Back then we were all hunter/gatherers.

If you were a vegetarian back in prehistoric times, that meant you were dead, because there were no concentrated sources of grains then. When the first seemingly smart human said, "Hey, we could put these seeds in the ground, pour water on them and take care of them," they didn't plant squash, beans and tomatoes; they planted cereal grains. So literally, in geological time, almost in the blink of an eye, human beings had this huge surplus of carbohydrates. It can be argued quite successfully by anthropologists that what happened with the dawn of the agricultural age and the culturing of cereal grains is that humans' bones got weaker, their bones got softer, feet got weaker; they didn't live as long – they had more diseases that started developing. Whereas the hunter/gatherer lifestyle was high protein, low carb, and lots of exercise.

That's just basic common sense. I'm not saying you shouldn't eat any carbohydrates. The two grains I actually recommend are quinoa and millet because they're higher protein, and they don't have as high of a glycemic index. They don't spike the blood sugar up like wheat and corn, and most wheat and corn today has been genetically modified many times over. So in general, I recommend, say, a Paleo diet, or higher protein/lower carb diet with higher amounts of healthy fat. This is similar to the Atkins Stage One diet. But with a diet like this you have to drink plenty of liquids to flush your kidneys, and you need some exercise.

Use a Mini-Trampoline for Bone Density Improvement? – Absolutely!

Although I don't present much about exercise in this book, I wanted to at least include this portion, because all of these components go together to create balance. I don't happen to believe in strenuous exercise, but just walking is of tremendous benefit to human beings. I also highly recommend to my patients that they invest in a mini-trampoline, because it really helps keep the bones dense; it pumps the lymphatic fluid around, and your immune system is a large part of the lymphatic system, not to mention the drainage capacity to get excess weight out of your body through the lymphatic system. Please note: I don't recommend they do big jumping routines on it, but more like what I call "giggling" – where you stand on it, and gently go up and down without your feet ever leaving the surface of the trampoline - almost a vibrational give-and-take. When I suggest getting a mini-tramp, almost everybody says, "I used to have one of those, but I don't know what I did with it…"

The thing with bone density is this - every time you're jumping or going up and down, you go to the bottom and get pushed back up again, then your whole body experiences more than one gravity of pull. Just for that moment. And your body will adapt to physical stresses it's put under all the time, just like it would if you carried a 30 pound pack on your back every day - your bone density would increase to adapt to that weight. You can get the same effect jumping up and down, doing jumping jacks or jumping rope on a concrete floor, but you'll destroy your ankles and your hips. Whereas when you're on a mini-trampoline, spring suspension protects your joints, and you can still get the benefit of gravity pulling on you. So I tell my patients, just 5 minutes in the morning and again in the evening can really benefit you physically.

The Ketogenic Diet

Back to diet - specifically with cancer, what I recommend is called a Ketogenic diet. There is a Ph.D. named Thomas Seyfried, who used to work in the lab at Yale; he's currently at Boston College. I mentioned him earlier on in the book. He expanded upon Dr. Warburg's work – and again, his book is titled *Cancer as a Metabolic Disease: On the Origin, Management and Prevention of Cancer*. It's an excellent book; he marvels at the fact that every doctor is taught about anaerobic metabolism and what it takes for it to prosper. Yet what boggles my mind is that they forget that in their training, and thereby do their patients a huge disservice. Seyfried has actually cured brain tumors in mice strictly with a Ketogenic diet and oxidative treatment with hyperbaric oxygen.

Hyperbaric oxygen therapy creates a large amount of free radicals within one's system. Hyperbaric treatments can include some risky factors, so we don't offer it at RIMC. We do incorporate five other oxidative therapies that will bring about the same positive results. I'll elaborate on the basics of this a bit.

Normal healthy cells have metabolic mechanisms to deal with free radicals and neutralize them through antioxidants. There are several ways to introduce antioxidants into one's system, for example, Vitamin C, Vitamin E and Vitamin A. This is why you'll find that the Ketogenic Diet regimen included below has blueberries, raspberries and strawberries, because they're packed with antioxidants and contain somewhat less of a sugar ratio than oranges or peaches, for example.

Cancer cells never deal with free radicals due to their anaerobic nature, which again, burn sugar without using oxygen, so no free radicals are created within them. On the other hand, the mitochondria within the body's normal cells burn sugar with oxygen and are always creating a certain amount of free radicals. These cells have developed the mechanism to deal with free radicals, but cancer cells have not evolved to a point where they can do so. As you'll discover in Chapter 6, which deals with the therapies we provide, one of the effects of implementing the various oxidative treatments offered at RIMC is to create an excess of free radicals.

It's interesting to note that the older, cheaper chemo drugs were designed to create free radicals. So they knew back then that free radicals would kill cancer cells. By getting our patients into a good state of ketosis, it makes the IPT and other oxidative therapies that we use at the clinic even more effective.

One recent study, which elaborates on the Ketogenic diet, occurred at UCLA. You can read about it in detail on a website called Pubmed.gov. This is a source that doctors around the world go to in order to learn about the latest research in medicine, because it publishes all global medical journals. If you want to read the UCLA article in its entirety, just go to Pubmed.gov and search "ketogenic diet."

This study goes into detail about the protocol for conventional chemo treatment, which begins with getting an I.V. infusion followed by a 3-week waiting period. Depending upon the results, at that time they repeat the infusion. They discovered that if patients would fast for two days before the infusion as well as on the day they received it, and additionally fasted for two days after the infusion, 99 percent of the bad effects of any of the chemos disappeared. The key to understanding these results is to know that fasting puts you into ketosis. This is the crux of the newer research showing that a Ketogenic diet definitely benefits cancer treatment.

Even though we don't offer hyperbaric oxygen treatments, the other oxidative treatments we use plus the Ketogenic diet cause the same positive results with fewer risks. If you'd like more details on hyperbaric treatment, or any of the other modalities mentioned in this book, please feel free to get in touch with us at RIMC.

Strangely enough, a Ketogenic diet consists of higher protein, higher healthy fats, and very low carbs. There are many parallels to the current fad called the Paleo Diet. The Ketogenic diet was originally developed to treat children with intractable seizures back in the 1960s. It does help them, but you have to be far more meticulous when you're treating children with seizures than you do with adult cancer patients.

What the word Ketogenic means, obviously, is that it generates ketone bodies; the brain is capable of switching its metabolism to burn ketones for energy and continuing to function. But cancer cannot make that switch. It has to burn simple sugars. So by limiting your sugar intake, and keeping your blood sugar at a minimal rate – in the lower part of normal – you can start to inhibit the cancer, but you cannot cure your cancer by not eating sugar. However, you can make it more susceptible to whatever other therapies you are using or applying if you are limiting your sugar and burning ketones. That's why I recommend a Ketogenic diet.

More and more studies are emerging which show what positive results/benefits a Ketogenic diet brings about, including (but not limited to) weight loss, cancer, Alzheimer's, help for those who deal with seizures, Parkinson's disease, Multiple Sclerosis and any neurological disease. Scientific medical proof on how it creates so many beneficial results to such a wide demographic is beyond exciting.

Immediately below is a copy of a document I give to all attendees of Boot Camp. It primarily concerns the Ketogenic Diet, which is outlined in detail afterward.

Anti-Cancer KETOGENIC Diet as Part of Therapy at RIMC

Dr. Bob says: "Extremely Important!!!"

I am writing this document because I cannot emphasize enough how important it is for you to follow our dietary guidelines. There are many opinions "out there" about what is good to eat and not good to eat for a person with cancer. There is only ONE diet that has been scientifically proven (repeatedly) to have weakening and killing effects on cancer cells. That diet is the Ketogenic diet.

This diet is not difficult to follow but it is likely very different from the diet you have been eating. RIMC will provide you with very specific guidelines to enable you to "stick to it." Any cheating will be your choice but will most definitely be detrimental to the possibility of overcoming this disease. In short, the Ketogenic diet consists of an increased amount of protein and (healthy) fats with very limited (to no) carbohydrates. The important thing to clearly understand is that ALL carbohydrates turn into sugar in your body.

Tumor cells thrive on sugar and cannot use any other kinds of fuel. Proteins and fats stimulate the formation of what are called "ketone bodies." All normal cells (most especially the brain cells) are capable of thriving on ketones. All other cells in your body can use ketones as fuel. Cancer cells require simple sugars on a moment-by-moment basis or they weaken. Research has proven if you can stay in ketosis with a relatively lower blood sugar, it weakens the cancer cells to the point that all of our other therapies have a much greater chance of eliminating them. I say again, I cannot emphasize enough how important this is! You are in a fight for your life and I am giving you a tool that has proven to help in that fight. It is in your hands. We will give you the skills and the information, but it is up to you to use the tool.

Ketogenic Journal: You will be asked to measure your blood sugar and blood ketones 3 times per day and keep a written record of the results. You will also be asked to record all the food you consume and the time you do so. These records will be extremely important to determine if you are staying in "ketosis" and if any food choices cause you to come out of it. Everyone is different in regards to ketosis. Certain foods may be okay for one person but not for another. This is the reason you need to keep an accurate food diary, Eventually you will know which foods are particular to your metabolism and ketosis.

*****

Here is the Ketogenic Diet Plan that I share with my patients:

KETOGENIC DIET

Goal: Force the body into ketosis. Ketosis is the result of the metabolic process of burning fat and protein for energy instead of carbohydrates. This blocks the ability of the cancer cells to produce energy from glycolysis (anaerobic metabolism).

NOTE: During Boot Camp, we'll be measuring the ketones in a patient's blood. If they are not in the right range/stage of ketosis, we'll endeavor to find out why. But it is non-negotiable – you must follow the Ketogenic diet in order for the other therapies we offer to be most effective.

I find it so interesting that people will argue about altering their diet, making excuses as to why they can't make changes, or using holidays or special occasions as a rationalization like, "It's too hard to eat that way when I'll be at a gathering where they're serving barbeque and other goodies." My answer is, "Too bad! Do you want to heal this or don't you?"

Sometimes they just tell me, "Oh, I don't know if I could stick with the Ketogenic diet." My response to this is, "I have a statement and a question for you. The question is, "If I had a tool or a treatment, or a weapon, if you will, that I could put in your hands that would kill your cancer, would you be interested in using that?" Of course, the response is a resounding, "Yes!" Then the statement that goes along with that question is, "The Ketogenic diet is that weapon, and it is that important. So don't tell me you can't do it – if you say you can't do it, then I question whether you want to survive this disease."

Because we provide recipes along with the Ketogenic diet, you needn't feel like you're being deprived of every "goodie" you love. For instance, there's a recipe for "Mock Mac & Cheese" that uses steamed cauliflower and is very tasty. So there are ways to make alternative choices to your old meal habits that will allow you to stay in ketosis.

Bear in mind – the easiest way for somebody to be kicked out of ketosis is to eat sugar. So it's critical that you avoid it at all costs. Okay – on with the specifics of the Ketogenic Diet!

Allowed: At least 6 ounces of fat and protein foods: grass-fed organic beef, poultry, wild-caught fish and shellfish, organic eggs, organic cottage cheese, kefir, sour cream, yogurt, butter 3 to 4 times per day.

It's allowed to have ¼ cup of organic brown, unprocessed rice or quinoa or millet one time per day with these proteins. Quinoa and millet are preferred over brown rice. Feel free to add spices and flavoring.

One lemon per day is also recommended.

Green leafy vegetables (except iceberg lettuce) have abundant anti-cancer properties and are filling, so eat as many green veggies as you like. Try sautéing with garlic for added flavor.

Alcohol: One glass of good quality red wine per day is allowed. Any other alcohol is strictly prohibited.

Prohibited: Processed sugars, starchy based foods such as potatoes, beans, corn, white rice, and pasta. Also all processed grain products such as pastries and breads. No cheeses except cottage cheese, and that only in small amounts (1/4 cup).

Liquids: WATER, herbal teas, fresh-made lemonade with Stevia, and V8 juices are all allowed.

1 to 2 cups of organic coffee are allowed, only if consumed within 30 minutes of brewing, because after that, it becomes acidic.

You are allowed to have a little organic heavy whipping cream in your fresh brewed coffee.

Oils: 4 to 6 tablespoons of organic butter (ghee is preferred), olive oil, organic hemp oil, grape seed oil, coconut oil, or coconut cream daily. Coconut oil, butter and grape seed oil are the best ones to cook with. Hemp oil and olive oil, on the other hand, should not be cooked with. You can eat coconut cream directly like a pudding if it appeals to you.

More recipes are available at tropicaltraditions.com

Coconut oil is solid at room temperature, so it must be warmed to liquefy.

Sweeteners: Stevia is the only sweetener allowed.

That's the essential Ketogenic Diet, and it is definitely an integral part of the therapies we do at RIMC. We consider it to be one of the pillars of the whole program we offer/teach.

There are a few additions I recommend just below.

Recommended Fruits and Types of Blenders

This diet includes some fruits. Normally you hear, "Oh, you need lots of fruits and vegetables," but what I prefer to say is, "What you really need is lots of vegetables, non-starchy vegetables, and a little bit of fruit because of the sugar." The types of fruit that I recommend most highly are blueberries, raspberries, strawberries and pomegranate because of the high ratio of antioxidants along with the lower sugar content. I highly recommend that people use a "Nutribullet." With this type of blender, you blend up everything, so you must use organic foods. Either a Nutribullet or a Vitamix blender will blend the whole vegetable. That way you get the fiber; otherwise much of the nutrition ends up going out with the pulp when you use other types of juicers. You have pulp left over then that you can either use in cooking, or maybe feed to your chickens or earthworms or whatever, but you lose the benefit of the nutrition in all that fresh pulp. So by using a Nutribullet or Vitamix, you personally are consuming that rich nutrition. You can also add things like hemp seed protein, chia seeds, etc., so that you get protein in a smoothie, too.

With regard to non-starchy vegetables and the like, one of the things we do recommend is tea. Specifically using it as part of the liquid added to the Nutribullet smoothies. Here's the combination of liquid:

- One-third aloe vera juice
- One-third unsweetened cranberry juice
- One-third parsley tea

The reason for the parsley tea is that it stimulates the kidneys. It's a natural diuretic, and of course, the kidneys are one of the major pathways for excretion of waste products, so we want to keep that open and flowing. Parsley is also high in potassium.

As far as actual veggies are concerned, cucumbers also have a natural diuretic quality, as well as celery and peppers – green peppers, yellow peppers, red peppers. Additionally, any of the other non-starchy vegetables are great. Avocados are excellent because of their great fat content. Avocados are great fat. Beets are wonderful when it comes to helping to cleanse the liver, and also I've seen them be very beneficial in boosting the hemoglobin level. Carrots should be consumed in moderation, because there's a lot of sugar in carrots. Green apple juice is good, so you can use half a green apple in a Nutribullet smoothie – no more than that, because you have to be concerned about the sugar in apples. Tomatoes are also very good.

On the Ketogenic diet plan above, you may have wondered about V8 juice, since it has a concentrated amount of sodium. They do make a low sodium version, of course, but if you can't find that at the store, you can just make a vegetable blend yourself, and naturally, making it fresh is best. But if you're on the road and don't have access to a blender, getting V8 Juice which is available in most stores is better than nothing.

The Importance of "Healthy Fats" – Omega 6 and Omega 3

When I'm discussing the Ketogenic diet with patients, I recommend higher fat intake but preface that with "healthy fat." One of those healthy fats is good organic hemp oil, because of the perfect ratio of Omega 6 and Omega 3 fatty acids. Our cell membranes are made up of a 2 to 1 ratio of Omega 6 to Omega 3, and to make good, healthy cell membranes, you need that very ratio. Most fats are only rated one way or the other, with the 3s or 6s rather than both.

The big fallacy that's out there right now is that fish oil and flax oil are healthy for you and so you should eat gobs of those; the problem with those is that flax oil and fish oil both are predominantly Omega 3s. Now, I'm not saying that either of those oils or Omega 3s are unhealthy – I'm saying that it's unhealthy to eat an overabundance of the 3s in relation to the 6s. You have to balance it out.

So you have to find out what's in the fats you're eating. If you want to eat those, I recommend organic hemp oil, coconut oil, grape-seed oil and olive oil, as well as avocados - they are really good.

I make a point to tell them that the most damaging fat is what's called "trans fat." Most people don't realize where trans fat originally came from; any product in the grocery store that has a fat in it, if it's stored on the shelf instead of a refrigerator – don't touch it. Because those fats are altered by bubbling hydrogen gas through them, and that creates a chemical bonding with the molecules in such a way that it turns it into a molecule that's pretty close to plastic.

If you don't know your history, you may be surprised to find out that this bubbling hydrogen gas into foodstuffs originated with Napoleon, of all people. He went to his quartermasters, wanting a substitute for butter, and they came up with margarine. They made it by bubbling hydrogen through vegetable oil. It looked like butter and they could add chemicals to it to make it taste like butter, but it isn't butter. There's an author named Brian Peskin who wrote a book called *The Hidden Story of Cancer.* In it, he talks about how the body treats these trans fats as normal fats, and incorporates them into cell membranes. But when a trans fat is deposited in the cell membrane, it ceases to allow oxygen to seep through it. And as Otto Warberg proved - if you cut the oxygen flow by 33 percent into any cell, it's going to flip over into anaerobic metabolism, which is cancer.

Mr. Peskin goes on to instruct people to go buy a tub of margarine at the grocery store. Then he says you should just open it up and put it on your kitchen counter; let it sit there, and see how long it takes before it "goes bad." And what's the definition of "going bad?" Basically, it means something else will start to eat it, like mold or fungus, or whatever. He goes on to say something along the lines of, "You'll find that tub of margarine can sit on your kitchen counter for up to a year without anything growing on it." That's because nothing else in nature wants to eat it, except stupid humans!

So fats are extremely important in treating cancer, because if you have people that are going through therapy, but they're eating canola oil or Twinkies off the shelf, and it's depositing these trans fats in their cell membranes, the cancer's going to be REAL happy and continue to grow.

Benefits of Fermented Foods

The other thing I highly recommend is fermented food, including dairy products such as kefir, yogurt, buttermilk, and sauerkraut. Especially in this country, we've really gotten away from the concept that in many cultures, a fermented food is a part of every meal because of the probiotic properties in them. I was astonished to learn something about fermented foods just a couple of years ago. I'm half-Polish, and grew up eating lots of sauerkraut. My grandparents had a big crock down in the basement where they made their own sauerkraut. So I was recently amazed to learn that the organism that makes sauerkraut when it ferments is the same organism that makes yogurt.

This is acidophilus, lactobacillus acidophilus. Of course there are a bunch of different strains of them, but that's the basic group. That's the reason why you read and hear from different sources, yogurt is good for your probiotics, and it's because of that organism. You can actually ferment any vegetable – pickles, cucumbers, carrots - the original pickles that were made were fermented just like sauerkraut, whereas most today are made with vinegar. Good organic apple cider vinegar is fermented, too, but anything that's canned like sauerkraut and pickles on the shelf that are not refrigerated until you open them, those don't have any probiotics in them anymore. In order for that to be the case today, they'd have to be refrigerated from the start. At Whole Foods, for example, you can now buy fresh sauerkraut in a refrigerated jar.

Also, I've started making my own buttermilk; I purchased some really good organic Bulgarian buttermilk and I ferment it, just like feeding a sourdough starter. I drink a small glass of it every morning. Lots of times on the weekend when I make breakfast, I'll make gluten-free pancakes or waffles and add ground-up almonds. I use buttermilk instead of water or milk for the liquid aspect of it. I think it would be healthy for people to get back to doing that on their own. But short of that, they could start to purchase these things at a place like Whole Foods.

In that refrigerated area you'll find Greek yogurt, Bulgarian yogurt – all kinds! Kombucha is another one. The reason those are all beneficial is because of the probiotics, which really help boost your immune system. They're starting to learn in conventional medicine how beneficial probiotics are for many things, not just restoring the population in the bowel. They can help actually treat infections, because they crowd out the bad bugs. And they're located throughout the body, not just in the bowel. So those are the general guidelines, dietary-wise that I recommend to people.

I believe it's important to have as broad a range of suggestions as possible, and not have to limit people to having such a strict guideline, like if you were to say, "Oh, no, no, no – you can only have half a teaspoon of that instead of a teaspoon," because as I mentioned, fanaticism in any regard is not beneficial.

Gluten-Free Foods

In general, I believe gluten-free products are better to lean toward. One major factor is the GMO foods these days. If you're going to have food sensitivities, food problems, gluten seems to be at the top of the list for a lot of people. The only people who really need gluten are vegetarians because it's a protein, so they want to get some of their protein from the grains. I know there are some vegetarians that want the gluten, but if you're going to develop any food sensitivities, gluten is right at the head of the line. It can trigger reactions in many people even if they don't have sensitivity. So I say if you can go the route of cutting out gluten or cutting down on your gluten intake, that's the best because there are many alternatives these days.

GMOs – Run the Other Way!

GMOs (Genetically Modified Organisms) are nothing short of a terrible idea. For obvious reasons they are detrimental to our own genetics, and the biggest contributing factor is because we don't even know what they're going to do once they enter our body. The counter argument that companies big into GMO production give is, "Oh, well, we've been genetically modifying plants for thousands of years." Simply not true. There's a difference between crossing two strains of wheat out in your field and genetically changing it in the lab so that it can tolerate Roundup. That's a whole different ball game. Some very revealing statistics are now showing up in studies being done that are more involved than the superficial crap that major GMO producers have done (which are short-term studies that conclude that they show no problem). These longer term studies that are more in depth have uncovered that consumption of GMOs not only starts doing damage to the lining of your small bowel, but also begins damaging your own genetics because of the gross abnormalities of lab produced GMOs.

Just as an interesting side note, I have come to believe that about 90 percent of the American population has leaky gut syndrome these days already. So when you add things like GMOs in the mix, look out.

Become a Voracious Label Reader

The biggest challenge I find patients have trouble with, dietary-wise, is Number 1 – they have to start paying attention in a big way. Many of them have never made a practice of carefully reading labels; they just blindly toss food into their cart, purchase it, and later consume it without a care or worry as to how it may affect them. Whenever they go grocery shopping, they don't think about whether there are Omega 6s in this, how much sugar is in that, or is there high fructose corn syrup in this other product? Is it organic, or not? Is it labeled GMO? To overcome cancer effectively, you must start reading labels and take more responsibility for your nutrition and health. Nobody else can do that for you.

Say Goodbye to Most of Your Favorite "Comfort Carbs"

Another big thing is giving up carbs, because like it or not, the bottom line is that carbs are the emotionally satisfying foods. For instance, when people get yelled at by their boss, they don't go home and eat a steak – they eat a bag of potato chips! And not only one, in many cases. The reason we reach for such highly processed carbs is because they produce an almost immediate sugar spike, which feels good and puts you in a mellower mood. It's astonishing when you realize that the sugar receptors in the brain are the same ones that are the receptors for cocaine. And guess who is well aware of this fact? Food manufacturers.

Alkaline vs. Acidic

I mention this subject in the Q & A chapter of the book, but want to delve deeper into it here.

Just to clarify, acidity does not cause cancer – it's actually the reverse in a sense. Acidity is a byproduct of cancer due to cancer's abnormal anaerobic metabolism – remember? It burns sugar without using oxygen. This creates one very large waste product, and that is lactic acid. Lactic acid is normal in a human body, but when it's created during anaerobic metabolism, much larger amounts of it are concentrated around the cancer cells, in their immediate environment. So it's the result of the cancer metabolism – not the cause of the cancer to begin with. In short, you cannot cure cancer by neutralizing the acidic environment.

It does make sense to try and keep healthy pH levels - pH is the scale or the measure of acid versus alkaline. A good rule of thumb is to take some measures to try to maintain a close to neutral pH in the human body. But this is also compounded or complicated by the fact that it's imperative for the pH of the blood in the body to swing back and forth between acid and alkaline throughout any given day in order to perform all the functions of the human body.

What I'm specifically referencing is the work of a doctor named Emanuel Revici, who was an M.D. in New York City. He was very well known for being successful at treating cancer. He was a Romanian physician and ran his own hospital, which his grateful patients purchased and then appointed him as the director. (If you'd like more information on his work, simply Google Emanuel Revici, or Revici Life Science Center of New York. You'll find a number of books written about him and his work).

Dr. Revici patented a hundred different medicines. However, he ran afoul of the AMA because these were natural remedies, and he had conflict with the political nature with the AMA; so they battled throughout his whole life. But Revici was the type of genius that only slept three hours a night; he would see patients during the day in his clinic and hospital, and then do research at night in his own lab.

Among his ideas, many of which I agree with, one of them is that if you look at any chemical process in nature, the value of the outcome of the chemical reaction will vary between two extremes around a neutral point. That's how the body maintains a balance. But the facts are, in physiology, if you are not acidic through part of the day, you cannot eliminate waste products. It's called catabolic metabolism – it means to tear down/break down tissue, and it is what helps us eliminate waste products from the body. Then when you swing into an alkaline pH, that's called anabolic metabolism, during which you build up antibodies that build and make hormones, therefore healing takes place during the anabolic process.

The concept that Dr. Revici propounded was that people's physiology should be acidic from 4 a.m. to 4 p.m., and that it should be alkaline from 4 p.m. to 4 a.m. I agree totally with that belief.

But there are many places online where you'll read that the more alkaline you are, the healthier you are. The problem with this line of thinking is that the one place where you have got to be heavily acidic all the time is in your stomach. If you do not have enough acid pH in your stomach, you cannot digest protein properly. So alkaline water machines and alkalinizing therapies actually interfere with the acid production in your stomach not only by breaking up the cycle of eliminating waste, but also rendering your body unable to properly digest protein.

It's very common for people in high alkaline states to have constipation problems and lung issues, because those are primary elimination areas of the body.

There are safe, healthy ways to move the body toward a balance point with this acid/alkaline process. One of those is drinking what's called "lemon water" – or taking doses of apple cider vinegar. While it seems counterintuitive to take an acid to create an alkaline environment, what happens when the body metabolizes or burns the product of what is in lemon juice or apple cider vinegar, it creates what's called a metabolic end product, or an "alkaline ash." The way to do this is to squeeze the juice of a half of a good organic lemon into a quart of water, and then consume that in the morning. Of course, this contains citric acid and ascorbic acid (Vitamin C) and morning is the time of day you're supposed to be acidic. By the time your body metabolizes the lemon water, it's the middle of the afternoon and it helps you swing into an alkaline pH.

It's the same with apple cider vinegar. I tell my patients to drink what I call "apple cider vinegar tea," because it's much more difficult to just take a swig of good old straight apple cider vinegar. To make the tea, put a couple of tablespoons of organic apple cider vinegar into a coffee cup or mug and add a little bit of stevia, and then fill it up with warm water, not hot water, because there are lots of good enzymes in true, fermented organic apple cider vinegar. Then you sip on that as a tea throughout the morning. This is essentially the same process as drinking lemon water – it helps with acidity, but then swings you into alkaline into the afternoon.

The Four Myths

The other thing I want to mention about diet is what I call the Four Myths. These are four typical things that people usually get told when they get diagnosed with cancer. The way I put it is, "Aunt Tilly calls 'em up and says, 'Oh, you're diagnosed with cancer? Well, then - you can't eat red meat, you can't drink coffee, you can't eat chocolate, and you can't drink red wine.'" But none of those four things are true.

I've already mentioned the best types of meat, which needs to be organic, grass-fed meat or wild meat, for obvious reasons.

The coffee - research has shown that good, clean organic coffee consumed within 20 to 30 minutes after brewing will have a very strong antioxidant effect, and caffeine can actually give a boost to your immune system as well as your alertness. So saying you can't have coffee is not true. But having commercial canned coffee that is not organic is not a good idea. It's also not a healthy practice to leave the pot on the stove and drink from it all day, which a lot of people do, or in the office where they have the coffeemaker in the break room that's always kept warm.

Next is chocolate. They have found in conventional research that when it comes to chocolate, the darker the better, because it has less sugar. The cacao actually has a very strong antioxidant effect. So good, organic dark chocolate is actually beneficial, in reasonable amounts, of course. There is a line of chocolate bars at Whole Foods called Lilly's, which contain no sugar– they sweeten them with Stevia. So dark chocolate is allowed within those parameters. Milk chocolate has too much sugar.

And then for red wine - I tell people, "I'm not suggesting you start drinking red wine if you don't drink alcohol, but if you really enjoy a nice glass of good, red wine at the end of the day, research has shown that the resveratrol in that red wine has an anti-aging effect, and a very strong antioxidant effect." So basically I tell my patients one or two glasses of good quality red wine a day is okay, but no cheap box wine!

So there you have the debunking of "Aunt Tilly's Four Myths."

Various Food Facts, and Food-Based Natural Supplements

There are many wonderful natural food-based supplements that can benefit someone's overall health, whether they have cancer or not. For example, I have black cumin seed oil stocked in my office, but I have not had that many patients on it yet. The big advantage of it that I have heard from some of my colleagues is it's supposed to have a suppressing effect on what are called "cancer stem cells." Cancer stem cells are the source of resistance cancer cells can develop to any given therapy, because most cancer therapies are designed to kill active cancer cells. Cancer stem cells are usually dormant unless the tumor perceives it's under threat of being totally wiped out, and then the stem cells get activated. And black cumin seed oil is supposed to be effective at suppressing the cancer stem cells.

I believe coconut oil is very beneficial. We use coconut in our IPT therapy – this is Insulin Potentiated Therapy. You'll read more about that in Chapter 6, which covers the various therapies we utilize. I'll touch upon it briefly here, too. When we drop people's blood sugar in order to administer things like laetrile, mistletoe and a low-dose ten percent chemo solution, then we reach a point where we have to raise their sugar level back up to normal. One of the ways we do that is with coconut water. Not in the I.V.s, just drinking it. Coconut water has a balance of electrolytes as well, but is natural, and not as severe as something like Gatorade to help achieve electrolyte balance. Many people now drink coconut water as opposed to other energy drinks that contain chemicals and highly processed sugar.

Aloe vera juice is wonderful for a number of reasons. The big benefit of it is that it's very soothing to the stomach lining and small bowel – it instigates healing to help correct digestive problems. I believe that most people, at least in the U.S. have some degree of what's called "leaky gut syndrome." I have this developing theory that leaky gut syndrome can be attributed to almost everything we eat in this country, because of how we've screwed up our digestive systems with chemicals and additives, GMOs…all the things that have taken us away from what really is a good, healthy diet. Then ultimately when you start getting leaky gut, you're impacting your immune system in some way, rarely in a positive way. Ultimately your immune system is supposed to help protect you from disease. But if it gets too far out of balance, it can even be the source of disease such as autoimmune diseases, allergies, and so on. Aloe vera juice isn't easy to drink straight, it doesn't taste all that great. But adding it into smoothies is an excellent way to consume it, usually by adding about a half-cup. If you wanted to take it in an eight-ounce glass of purified water, I'd recommend adding about four tablespoons.

Milk Substitutes

It's a well-known fact that humans are the only animals on the planet that continue to drink milk after childhood. Cow's milk is designed to be baby food, and it contains high quantities of what's called "growth factor." The last thing a cancer patient wants is growth factor. When it comes to dairy products in general, I tell people whole dairy products are a big no-no.

As a healthy alternative, I highly recommend almond milk, as well as coconut milk. Rice milk not so much, since rice is a carbohydrate.

I already mentioned that eating fermented foods as being excellent for digestive health. Part of the reasoning is that the fermentation process breaks down the growth factor proteins so they're much safer. Plus, those fermented dairy products such as yogurt, kefir and the like, provide probiotics, which are good for helping to heal leaky gut as well. So instead of telling my patients absolutely no dairy products of any kind, I tell them to stick with the fermented ones. However, speaking of strict no-nos, soy should be considered one of them – it's basically not good for anyone.

What About Water?

When it comes to my recommendation on water consumption, I used to say, "Half your body weight in ounces." That's been a standard rule of thumb in naturopathic medicine for a long time. But more recently, I think that's excessive. Moreover, I think it's an unobtainable quota for most people, because when you're talking about a 150-pound person, that's 75 ounces. 64

ounces is half a gallon, so 75 ounces a day, day after day, is a difficult goal to obtain, and it's debatable as to whether it's too much.

So I tell people in general, "you should be drinking enough good clean fluid, with water being the largest percentage of that, in order to make you have to urinate every three or four hours, minimum - during the day, of course. So you leave it up to the person unless, of course, there are mitigating factors about kidney function; then you would modify it. Same with someone with heart disease - bloating them up with so much water, half of their body weight in ounces – that's going to put a big strain on the heart as well. So I don't go with a standard amount across the board.

Water Purification

I feel the best water is distilled water because every water purification system other than distilling removes the toxins, waste and so on *from* the water. However, when you distill, you remove the *water* from the waste one molecule at a time. So you boil the water, make it into a vapor and then re-condense it through a condenser. The argument some people have against distilling is that it will deplete minerals from your body, which is true. But I say, Number One, it will deplete minerals, but it will deplete toxic as well as healthy minerals, which you want;

so Number Two, you must replace the minerals. You either replace them by taking a multivitamin, multi-mineral supplement, or via liquid minerals.

In my home we add liquid suspensions of minerals to each quart. We mostly keep our drinking and cooking water in mason jars, and then add liquid minerals into each jar, the healthy minerals. That way you're keeping the healthy minerals coming back into your body and getting rid of the toxic ones. This is the most pure water on the planet. Actually, rainwater is naturally distilled water.

You can purchase a distiller online; for example, a 3 to 4 quart countertop distiller will easily meet your water needs for the day, both for drinking and cooking. So you don't need some big system for your whole house. Something you do not want to do is to buy and consume distilled water in those soft, cloudy plastic jugs because they leach plastic out of the jug and into the water.

The other system that produces good, clean water is reverse osmosis (R.O.). The thing I have against reverse osmosis is it takes three times the amount of water to purify what you wind up with as the end product. So it's a HUGE use of water to get a smaller amount of usable water. Especially in places like California and other states experiencing drought conditions,

R.O. uses a lot of water only to end up with a small amount of product. Distilling gets around that problem.

NOTE: *As of this book's initial printing (2016), I am working on a cookbook for cancer patients, as well as for others who simply wish to improve their overall health through better dietary regimens. Please refer to our website - renointegrative.com for the announcement of the cookbook's release.*

Chapter 6

Boot Camp & Various Therapies

Our three-week Boot Camp is 5 days a week for 3 weeks, originated by Dr. Doug Brodie, the doctor I came to Reno to work with. I have continued with that same principle. That being said, there are some protocols used to treat cancer in clinics in this country as well as in Mexico, which also utilize the three-week time period. The concept that's vital to understand is that we never tell people the cancer will be cured within three weeks and it'll be gone.

There's a concept called a "critical threshold" and that means time enough to start the healing process. That's what we view the three-week time period as, and then instruct them on how to continue with different therapies at home. Additionally, we have our patients return to our clinic for three to five days once a month after the end of Boot Camp, until we can verify that the cancer is resolved.

A pic-line or a port is necessary in order to participate in the Boot Camp. A pic-line is a plastic catheter placed in a vein in the arm so that it reaches inside – the tip of the catheter sits in the largest vein in the body, right outside of the heart. A port is an actual silicone diaphragm over the top of a stainless steel chamber that has the same kind of catheter running out of it, so the tip of the catheter is put into the largest vein in the body. The reason for both of these catheter placements is that some of the I.V.s (intravenous therapies) that we use are very irritating to the lining of the smaller veins. By putting them through a pic-line or a port, it deposits the substances in the largest vein so it can be the most diluted by the blood, and therefore it does not irritate the lining of the larger vessel. An important thing for people to understand is that the placement of the pic-line or the port – for the most part, for our patients - will be covered by their medical insurance. Now, the advantages and disadvantages of the pic-line versus the port are as follows:

1) A pic-line is placed by a radiologist in a clinic, using local anesthetic or numbing medicine. The patient is still awake during the whole process; they don't get put to sleep. The advantages of the pic-line are: it's easier to put in, it's less expensive, and after it's in, the majority of the injections go through a valve on the end of this tube that is on the outside of the body in the arm. The disadvantage of the pic-line is that it can only stay in for a maximum of 6 months, and it has to be flushed once a week with an anticoagulant medicine to keep it from clotting shut.

2) The advantage of the port is that once it's put in, it can stay in place for years; this is because its silicone domed diaphragm chamber is placed under the skin during a surgical procedure, and sutured in place. Then the skin is sewn shut over the top of that and the port is accessed by using a special kind of needle that goes through the skin and through the silicone diaphragm. Now, the disadvantage of the port is it is about 5 or 6 times more expensive, because the patient has to be put to sleep and a surgeon has to place the port and then sew the skin back shut. But once it's in, the advantage is it can stay in for a few years if taken care of properly.

So having a pic-line or a port is a requirement for Boot Camp, and generally full dose chemo treatment for cancer requires a port placement.

Therapies

The initial overview statement I give my patients is, "Our therapies consist of protocols that actually attack and kill cancer cells as well as therapies that strengthen the immune system. Some of the other therapies de-cloak the cancer or make the immune system able to find the cancer even where it's hiding in the body." It's important to realize that there's integration between all the different therapies in the protocol, and that's why it works as well as it does. A number of people have come in saying, "Well, I just want to do this, or that…" but it doesn't work nearly as well as the whole integrative program. It's a synergistic process.

IPT Therapy

One of our biggest tools is Insulin Potentiated Therapy, or I.P.T. It was first developed in Mexico in the 1920s. As a cancer therapy, it is based on the proven fact that all cancer cells utilize a form of metabolism, or energy production, called anaerobic metabolism. This means that they burn sugar without using oxygen, as discussed earlier in this book.

By using intravenous insulin, we can put the cancer cells into a position where they are literally starving for sugar to the point that they get desperate and do what's called "opening up their cell membrane" in order to try to snag any sugar coming through the blood. When they do that, it creates a blood sugar level that's not good for cancer cells, but it's not harming normal cells, because they have a much lower need for sugar. Then we give a tiny dose of sugar that's mixed with different components that are delivered more specifically to the cancer cells, because of this greater need for sugar. A number of these components are laetrile, mistletoe, and salicinium, and we can talk about each of these in detail. But we also do use chemo drugs; although they are standard chemo drugs, we only use 10 percent of the full dose. These are delivered with this dose of sugar so that it is taken up much more completely by the cancer cells than by normal cells. This treatment is given twice a week during the three-week Boot Camp period.

I believe IPT is more effective than full dose chemo, even though the dose is 90 percent less. Because of this, we have 90 percent less bad effects from the chemo drugs as well. It's more effective because we're specifically targeting the cancer cells.

NOTE: I'm very excited to report that RIMC is on the cutting edge when it comes to the following: By utilizing a meter to determine if a patient's blood has enough ketones to render the IPT treatments most effective, we can kick the blood sugar into the right range by using protein and fat. We're calling it "Ketotic IPT" and right now, we're the only alternative cancer treatment facility using this method.

The next thing we do is called UBI - ultraviolet blood irradiation. We use ultraviolet light to irradiate the blood sample, and ultraviolet light is deadly to all viruses, most bacteria, and all cancer cells. This is done immediately after each IPT treatment.

Another therapy that we combine with the ultraviolet light is called oxidative therapy. It's the use of ozone gas and hydrogen peroxide, high dose intravenous Vitamin C, and breathing medical grade oxygen to raise the blood levels of oxygen, because it's harmful to these cancer cells due to their anaerobic metabolism (not using oxygen). So the different oxidative therapies are combined with the whole protocol in a very specific order.

The next thing that we utilize is called salicinium, which can be termed a "fake sugar." This is because it fools the cancer cells into thinking it's a sugar molecule, when in fact, it's delivered what's called a benzaldehyde ring, (a 6 carbon benzaldehyde ring). When this enters the cancer cell, it interferes with the energy production pathway in such a way that it kills cancer cells. On a cellular level, the way I put it to patients is, "The cell cannot skip breakfast and have a bigger lunch like we can. It needs to have a steady supply of energy production." If that energy production is cut off for any reason, even for a moment, that cell dies. That's what this salicinium does; it blocks the energy pathway inside the cancer cell.

Immune Therapies

The immune therapies are designed to:
1) Strengthen the immune system, and

2) Give it the specific tools it needs to identify the cancer cells in such a way that it will start attacking the cancer cells and killing them.

This is the reason why it is such bad therapy to use treatments that harm the immune system, because in conventional chemotherapy and radiation, many times the immune system is utterly destroyed, so it is helpless if the cancer recurs.

The first thing we do is to continue to use specific vitamin and mineral I.V. formulas that Dr. Brodie developed over the course of thirty years. Those are given on a regular schedule throughout Boot Camp. Then we also start supplements with our patients that boost the T cell count and the macrophage count. The T lymphocytes and the macrophage cells are white blood cells in the human body whose job it is to kill abnormal cells, which are the cancer cells. There are specific oral supplements that can be used to boost the number of these cells.

Then we utilize a compound called GcMAF – the MAF stands for "Macrophage Activating Factor." Here's the reason why, and what actually take place. When a normal cell flips over and goes into anaerobic metabolism, the metabolism of cancer – at the same time, it also begins producing an enzyme called nagalase. Nagalase turns off the macrophage cells, which are supposed to protect you from cancer. So this is a way the cancer has of hiding from the immune system, or what I call "cloaking."

The GcMAF is a tiny injection that injects this macrophage-activating factor back into the body to turn those macrophage cells back on again so they can detect the abnormal cancer cells. A Dr. Yamamoto in Philadelphia, Pennsylvania did the research on developing and proving this in the 1990s and into the 2000s. Dr. Yamamoto has since moved back to Japan, and we get our GcMAF from the company that he works with there. GcMAF is an injection that is administered just under the skin, two times per week.

TCRP is another type of immune therapy that can be termed "dendritic cell vaccine." It's a process that we use to concentrate these T cells and macrophage cells out of a person's blood; then we incubate them overnight in an incubator at what is a fever temperature in the human body. This process stimulates these cells to start producing what's called "heat shock protein." Heat shock protein has two functions – they can actually enable the T cells and the macrophages to kill cancer cells, and in addition, they can also function as messengers to tell the immune system where to go to find these cancer cells. This treatment is done one time per week, and when it is administered it's given in conjunction with the GcMAF.

There are a couple of other things that we use that can be categorized as apoptosis enhancement. I've described apoptosis earlier in the book, but just to recap - the thing to understand is that every single one of our normal cells has a DNA program contained within the mitochondria, which is essentially a self-destruction or self-suicide program. Now, the mitochondria are the energy furnaces found in every single cell. The concept is if that cell is harmed beyond the ability to heal, whether it's chemical, electrical or physical, in normal circumstances, this apoptosis program is triggered and the cell will commit suicide.

The example I give patients is that's why your kidneys stopped growing when they reached adult size. The mitochondria get turned off in a cell when it switches over into anaerobic metabolism, so this apoptosis program is turned off and that's why cancer cells grow out of control and ultimately cause what they cause. But there are some compounds that have been shown to reignite these mitochondria and the apoptosis program; compounds that reignite the mitochondria long enough to activate or reactivate the apoptosis program so that the cancer cell determines its own abnormality or dysfunctionality, and the apoptosis program will cause the cell to die. So in essence, once the cancer cell is de-cloaked you need to have a way of attacking it. One of the ways to do this is to stimulate apoptosis.

One of the compounds that reactivates the apoptosis is called DCA or dichloroacetate. By the way, this work was done at the University of Alberta in Canada, up to and including human trials, where they showed that DCA administration triggered apoptosis in these abnormal cells.

The second compound that we use is butyrex, and butyrex is the salt of butyric acid. Butyric acid is what's contained in cottage cheese and sour cream. And the salt of this butyric acid has been shown to help re-stimulate apoptosis. So we use both of these compounds in capsule form, they're an oral therapy.

The other aspect that I haven't mentioned is a drainage protocol that's done in a coordinated fashion throughout the three-week Boot Camp. Drainage, of course, is the term for all the systems in the body that are designed to detox and get waste out of the body, get it removed. So we have a number of treatments that we have a therapist apply to help the patient get rid of the waste products from the breakdown of the tumor cells. If the person cannot drain the waste products, it's very possible for the tumor to be shrinking, but the person is feeling worse and getting sicker. So we use tools such as the Biomat, which uses heated amethyst crystals that radiate far infrared heat waves. The mat contains amethyst crystals that get heated up, and then the person lies on the mat along with a separate mat that is laid on top of them for a set period of time. These far infrared heat waves penetrate six to seven inches into the body, so that's much deeper than a regular heating pad or hot water bottle. The concept to remember is not only does this open up the lymphatic pathways to help the lymph system drain off this waste, but it's also a fact that cancer cells, as a general rule, cannot stand extra heat. They do not have a heat dissipation process like our normal cells do. So as the heat builds up in the body, it can also be called hyperthermia, or high temperature therapy.

We have a number of other tools incorporated into our detoxification program that are designed to help open the drainage channels to help eliminate the waste that is the product of killing the cancer.

You can read more details about these various therapies on our website - www.renointegrative.com

Grounding/Earthing

There is a concept called grounding or "earthing" that I'd like to touch upon. It involves establishing a grounding effect between your body and the earth. Dating back to man's early history, when we first went barefoot and then eventually moved into wearing leather-soled footwear, we still were connected electrically to the planet whenever we walked outdoors. In other words, we are able to derive electrons from the earth because it has an electrical charge. So today, grounding is the concept of walking barefoot on wet grass or wet ground to establish this connection. The vast majority of modern day footwear is made of nonconductive material. (That's why they insulate electrical terminals with rubber, since it does not conduct electricity). Most shoes today are made from spongy foam-like synthetic materials very similar to rubber, if not rubber itself; this insulates you away from the earth.

You can learn much more about this by visiting www.earthing.com, but I'll give a bit of explanation, because I believe it's a viable form of therapy, not just for cancer patients, but everyone. They offer various apparatuses on this website - from a metallicized bed sheet to an actual electrode that is worn with an elastic band around the ankle or wrist; then there is a wire that runs from that and connects into the round grounding hole in every electrical outlet in a modern home. There's a tool that you plug into each outlet to establish whether it's properly grounded to the earth (that's what the grounding line is for). They've done extensive research that proves the benefits of regular grounding. If intrigued by this, visit earthing.com for complete details.

There is an option to achieve the same effect that doesn't involve purchasing any special equipment. You can easily integrate some grounding, or earthing, into your regular routine by simply walking barefoot on the grass (preferably wet grass, so just after watering is an ideal time) on a daily basis. Be aware of your surroundings while doing so, especially if you live in an area where snakes, scorpions or other poisonous critters make their home.

Another way to achieve the same effect would be to walk barefoot along the beach, preferably in wet sand. It feels wonderful, may stir up some pleasant childhood memories of being more in tune with our planet, and it's actually a great way to clear your mind, feel more centered and at peace. Enjoy!

Chapter 7
Energy Medicine

Just below is an article written by Dr. Bob about the benefits of energy medicine. Following that article is more detailed information about the types of energy medicine offered by Reno Integrative Medical Center.

***

Energy Medicine - The Evidence Continues to Mount!
By Robert A. Eslinger, D.O., H.M.D., DAAIM

It is ironic that our nearly 3 trillion dollar medical system actually uses some of the most sophisticated diagnostic equipment available in the world today to detect and measure energies and frequencies in the body.

You have probably heard of most of these. They include MRI's, PET scans, Cat scans, EEG's, EKG's, ultrasound devices and more.

Our medical system diagnoses the body energetically with modern physics (Quantum Field Theory), and then treats it with drugs and surgery (matter based Newtonian Mechanics) like a biological machine. What is wrong with this picture!?!

Quantum field theory has completely rewritten the book of science at the most fundamental level. However, modern biology and medicine continue to reference from a moldy, outdated book based on Newtonian science.

If you think "reality" is the world you can see, hear, taste, smell and touch it is time to re-evaluate. If you think your body is solid and governed by fixed laws, think again. That world just does not exist! It is an illusion.

The first thing to understand is that fields are the essential elements in nature (not particles). The first fields to be studied were the electric and magnetic fields. James Maxwell unified these into electromagnetic fields.

Quantum field theory essentially explains that we are not a huge number of particles held together by an energy field. Our bodies are actually formed primarily of energy and information fields.

Perhaps you are thinking this is a bunch of new age talk with no real science to back this up. Well, think again. The human bio-energetic holographic body is measurable up to 15 feet off the body surface. This has been scientifically proven.

So the shift is here. It is happening right now. Newtonian physics and the primacy of matter is a thing of the past. The human body is primarily energy and information. There are ways to measure it and find distortions (imbalances) in it and there are tools to help restore the balance.

Oschman, James, *Energy Medicine: The Scientific Basis*, Elsevier Limited 2000

Meyers, Bryant A., *PEMF (Pulsed Electromagnetic Field Therapy)- The 5th Element of Health*, Balboa Press 2014

****

What follows is more information about the various types of energy medicine offered by Reno Integrative Medical Center:

When dealing with the energetic medicine aspect of things, we're addressing not only the person's physical body, but the body field as well. By this I mean the field around the body, and this is not the aura. The aura is the etheric body. The body field is the sum total of all electrical and chemical activity going on in the body. By using the various energy systems we employ, we can find imbalances in the body field and correct them. The main systems we use for this purpose are the NES system, and the ZYTO system.

The ZYTO System

The first treatment technique we use is called a Zyto – Z-Y-T-O. If you wish, you can go online and find information at zyto.com, but essentially this is a computer program that allows us to communicate with a person's autonomic nervous system. Now, the thing to understand is that the autonomic nervous system is the other nervous system in all of our bodies.

I've touched upon it earlier in this book, but to briefly revisit it, it's the one that runs everything that's on automatic, like the heart rate and breathing rate - all the things we don't have to think about to have them happen. One of the things the autonomic nervous system controls is the electrical conductivity of the skin. So this equipment allows us to ask questions electronically of the autonomic nervous system, enabling us to detect if the autonomic nervous system thinks it is in harmony with what the body wants; and then to be able to utilize this equipment to develop specific remedies to help balance any imbalances that are found. That's called the Zyto system, and this is done in an office visit one time per week during the three-week Boot Camp.

NES

Then we have an additional piece of equipment that is part of what's called NES – N-E-S is the abbreviation for Neutri Energetic Systems. This computerized program uses quantum physics principles to detect imbalances in the body field, the whole body field. They call them distortions, or sometimes I call them imbalances in the human body field. And neshealth.com is the website for this. It's a system that was developed over the past 30 years by two men – one from England, one from Australia. It uses quantum physics principles to find what they call distortions in the human body field. Then there are specific liquid remedies that are put in water and drunk by the patient to correct these imbalances.

PEMF

There's also an electronic treatment that's called PEMF, and PEMF stands for Pulsed Electromagnetic Frequencies. You can Google PEMF and find that there are many systems out there right now using PEMFs to treat many conditions of the human body. But specifically we use them to correct these distortions in the human body field. The way I explain the whole concept of the body field to patients is, if you run an electric current through a copper wire, it creates a field around that wire; and this is a very similar concept with the body. The field interacts with the body and helps create the body, and the body also helps create the field. It's an interaction between the two things. So the concept is that by correcting these imbalances or distortions in the body field, ultimately it will lead to a correction in the body itself.

DR. BOB'S CONCLUSION

I hope this book has provided you with some information of which you were previously unaware.

I really wanted to dispel some myths, as well as to pull back the curtain to reveal some simple truths about cancer that can contribute to decreasing the fear around a cancer diagnosis.

In addition to practicing integrative medicine, I believe it's my mission to let people know that having cancer does not necessarily mean a death sentence, and that there is much cause for hope.

There is no such thing as "false hope" - that is a lie! And please remember - the time to give up hope is after you take your last breath!

It's my intention that this book will give you a sense of empowerment and a feeling that you do not have to accept the old worn out phrase - "your only choice is chemo, radiation and surgery." There are viable, powerful alternatives.

You don't have to accept my word for it. Do your own research...the truth is out there!

For further information contact Reno Integrative Medical Center, 6110 Plumas St., Ste. B, Reno, NV 89519, 775-829-1009, www.renointegrative.com

Tips for Caregivers

Hopefully, many caregivers as well as patients will read this book. They are integral to a patient's healing and well-being, and at RIMC we value their energy, love and their vital role in their loved one's life.

The biggest, most important tip for a cancer patient caregiver is to fully support the decisions of that patient for the kind of treatment he/she chooses. Most everyone agrees that we all have the basic right to choose what happens to our own body.

When a person is diagnosed with cancer, helplessness tends to be the most common emotion. Investigating choices and therapies should be an open-minded search for all available options. Whatever their ultimate decision, it should never be interfered with by a caregiver or their physician. I have seen this happen far too often. However, letting the patient know that you're there to do any necessary research that they may be unable to do themselves, and then to openly talk it over together provides a safe haven for them.

The most destructive thing I have seen patients face is antagonism and lack of support in choices they desire, in everything from diet to therapies to the location of those treatments from close friends, family members and worst of all, by closed-minded physicians.

I know that belief in one's choices is imperative to derive the maximum benefit from the chose therapies, whether those are conventional or integrative/alternative.

Anything less actually interferes with the healing.

The "Care & Feeding" of
Caregivers Themselves

Numerous studies have been conducted which show that caregivers tend to put themselves at the "bottom of the totem pole" when it comes to directing their energy as well as physical and emotional stamina. This is natural, and for the most part necessary in order for the patient's condition to improve. However, there's an old paradigm that advises along these lines – "If you don't take care of yourself, you won't have anything left over to give to others."

Here's another way to think of this: Before an airplane leaves the runway, the flight attendants give the typical instructional speech that most seasoned travelers essentially ignore. But wisdom can be found wherever you seek it, and this tip refers to the part of the attendant's speech about the oxygen masks.

They say something to this effect, "Should the oxygen masks fall down, be sure to first put one on…." Who? You, right? "Put yours on before assisting others." That makes a lot of sense. If you're not getting proper oxygen flowing to your brain and throughout your system, how can you possibly think straight and make good choices while helping others? So it's an excellent example to bear in mind when providing caregiving for others. The patient's needs come first, naturally. But please do the necessary self-care along the way – learn to recognize the signs when you're approaching a "burnout" point.

You may find yourself less patient with your patient for a variety of reasons. If you're not getting enough sleep, or are the only one on call 24/7, even if you're a superhero (you're not, okay?) you'll eventually reach a breaking point. And sleep deprivation only serves to amplify every little thing that you could otherwise deal with, no problem. So it's a good idea to seek out at least one other person to be on call to pitch in, if at all possible. Even if they can't give you a break for an entire day or two, that's okay. Someone who can spell you when you have to run errands, and your patient isn't well enough to accompany you, but cannot stay home alone is a very valuable person to have on your team. Someone who can come in at least once a week and attend to the patient's needs while you go out for a couple of hours to have dinner with a friend, go to a movie, go for a hike, get a massage, or maybe just take a blissful two to three hour nap, knowing that someone else is watchfully taking great care of your patient.

You'll find that simply doing some activity that will help you just clear your mind and rejuvenate so that when you're back on duty, you feel refreshed. You owe it not only to yourself, but also to your patient, to be at the top of your game as often as possible. So seek out other family members, neighbors, friends or professional home caregivers who can step in periodically and help out. You never know until you ask, and you'll find that quite often, people are more than willing to pitch in and be helpful.

If your budget can't accommodate professional home nurses or assistants, check out any volunteer organizations in your neighborhood. If you're a churchgoer, that is often an excellent place to seek volunteers. Do your homework early on, so that you outsmart and outmaneuver a breaking point.

It's ideal if you go on the Ketogenic diet along with your patient, especially if you're the one preparing meals (which is usually the case). You'll find it's a wonderful diet for everyone, and provides many benefits to all who follow it. That's the main reason it's suggested here, but it will also help avoid having other food and drink in the house that your patient can't have, and might wind up resenting seeing you consume.

It's a good idea to keep some favorite comedy DVDs handy, as well as music that you and the patient find relaxing and enjoyable. If you enjoy reading aloud, then some of your patient's favorite books should be handy. If you need to conserve your voice or would prefer, there are tons of great books on audio (www.audible.com, for example) that have been recorded by professional voice actors and keep the listener engaged and entertained. You can both enjoy those. If you have a shared hobby, then consider having an art therapy session once in awhile, or crocheting – wherever your talents and interests lead you.

If possible, go for scenic drives periodically for a change of venue, fresh air and beautiful vistas, which will stimulate the relaxation response in all who participate, and set the stage for maximum healing.

The main point here is that you participate in all of the positive activities you possibly can with your patient, but also know that you need and deserve an occasional break for some "me" time in order to help yourself stay cheerful, energized and in balance. Statistically, it's been shown that a number of caregivers wind up getting some type of physical ailment themselves if they don't make sure they're doing proper self-care. You may want to look into some support groups online or ones that might be held in your area, where you can talk out and learn from others some of the best ways to do your utmost for your loved one, while doing the necessary self-maintenance to stay at the top of your game.

And finally, to all caregivers - thank you and bless you for all you do. YOU are invaluable, and a key ingredient in the healing process.

BIBLIOGRAPHY

Please Note: This is not intended in any way to be a comprehensive bibliography about cancer (which would obviously be enormous!), but lists the books mentioned in *Outmaneuver Cancer*, as well as some others you may want to look into. You'll find that once you start learning more about alternate and integrative therapies, you'll be led to many resources to continue your discovery process. Happy Reading!

The Coconut Ketogenic Diet: Supercharge Your Metabolism, Revitalize Thyroid Function, and Lose Excess Weight, Dr. Bruce Fife

Cancer as a Metabolic Disease: On the Origin, Management and Prevention of Cancer Thomas Seyfried, PhD

Tripping Over the Truth: The Return of the Metabolic Theory of Cancer Illuminates a New and Hopeful Path to a Cure, Travis Christofferson

The Whistleblower: Confessions of a Healthcare Hit Man, Peter Rost, M.D.

The Truth About Drug Companies: How They Deceive Us and What to Do About It, Marcia Angell, M.D.

Anatomy of an Illness: As Perceived by the Patient, Norman Cousins

The Hidden Story of Cancer, Brian Peskin

Energy Medicine: The Scientific Basis, James L. Oschman, PhD

PEMF - The Fifth Element of Health: Learn Why Pulsed Electromagnetic Field (PEMF) Therapy Supercharges Your Health, Bryant A. Meyers

Defeat Cancer: 15 Doctors of Integrative and Naturopathic Medicine Tell You How, Connie Strasheim (NOTE: Dr. Bob contributed Chapter 8 of this book)

Changing Normal: How I Helped My Husband Beat Cancer, Marilu Henner – The former star of TV's *Taxi* eloquently shares how she worked with her husband to help him overcome cancer without chemotherapy or radiation.

E-books

Fight Cancer with a Ketogenic Diet- A New Method for Treating Cancer, Ellen Davis, M.S., www.ketogenic-diet-resource.com

** Google this to get the full benefit - *Get Started with the Ketogenic Diet - Moving Towards an Anticancer Life,* Miriam Kalamian, EdM, MS, CNS